MEDICINE MOVES TO THE MALL

CENTER BOOKS ON SPACE, PLACE, AND TIME

George F. Thompson, *Series Founder and Director*

Published in cooperation with the Center for American Places
SANTA FE, NEW MEXICO, AND HARRISONBURG, VIRGINIA

MEDICINE MOVES TO THE MALL

David Charles Sloane & Beverlie Conant Sloane

The Johns Hopkins University Press   Baltimore & London

The Johns Hopkins University Press
2715 North Charles Street
Baltimore, Maryland 21218-4363
www.press.jhu.edu

Library of Congress Cataloging-in-Publication Data

Sloane, David Charles.
  Medicine moves to the mall / David Charles Sloane and Beverlie Conant
Sloane.—1st ed.
        p. cm. — (Center books on space, place, and time)
Includes bibliographical references and index.
  ISBN 0-8018-7064-X (hbk. : alk. paper)
  1. Social medicine.   2. Medical care—Social aspects.   3. Medicine—Social
aspects.   4. Medicine—Miscellanea.   I. Sloane, Beverlie Conant.   II. Title.
III. Series.
RA418 .S576 2002
362.1'042—dc21
2001008645

A catalog record for this book is available from the British Library.

To our parents,

Jack and Rosemary, Ralph and Audrey,

with all our love

Contents

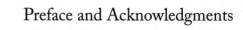

Preface and Acknowledgments

T his short book has been long in the making. We first started thinking about it and taking photographs for it in the early 1990s. At that time we were living in Hanover, New Hampshire, and watching as the new Dartmouth-Hitchcock Medical Center rose out of the forest to replace the quaint but outmoded Mary Hitchcock Hospital. The mall design of the new structure inspired this study.

Later, after moving to Los Angeles, we were struck by how rapidly the healthcare landscape there was being transformed. Not only were new designs being applied to the region's ambulatory care and specialty facilities, but the automobile-centered urban form of the city provided an ideal setting for the proliferation of what we came to call mini-mall medicine.

Although these two sites played important roles in the story we are going to tell, they are only representative of national, even international, trends that this book describes and analyzes. After each presentation that we have given on this topic, audience members have responded with evidence from their cities and towns. Whether in Chicago or Philadelphia, Boston or Tucson, in Bradenton, Florida, or Albany, New York, medicine is moving into the mall everywhere.

COLLEAGUES AND STUDENTS from our days at Dartmouth and in Los Angeles have provided keen insights, helpful research, criticism, and suggestions. We want to thank especially, Annmarie Adams, Alex Bontemps, Gert Brieger, Ralph Conant, Greg Hise, and Dell Upton, each of whom read the entire manuscript and provided us with a wealth of suggestions for improvement. Marshall Winn gave us a consumer perspective at a critical moment. Deepak Bahl, Alan Brandt, Margaret Crawford, Michael Dear, Elizabeth Gearin, Paul Groth, Alexis Jetter, Richard Longstreth, and Annelise Orleck helped gather materials and think through the study's issues.

Todd Gish and Ashwani Vasishth aided with both the research and the drawings that appear in the galleries.

We were fortunate to get feedback on the study's issues from colleagues who participated in seminars and lectures held by Dartmouth College's History Department Seminar, Dartmouth Medical School, the University of Southern California Geography Colloquium, and the USC planning school's History, Theory and Design Workshop and Institute of Civic Enterprise seminar.

The faculty and staff of the School of Policy, Planning, and Development at USC have been unfailingly supportive of our research. We particularly thank Deans Peter Gordon, Edward Blakely, Genevieve Giuliano, Bob Biller, and Daniel Mazmanian for their support. Melissa Azarcon, Linda Bakabak, Jung Kim, Anna Sai, Nina Tibayan, and other staff members have been generous with their time and help.

We would like to thank the National Endowment for the Humanities, the Lusk Center for Real Estate Development, and the John Randolph Haynes and Dora Haynes Foundation for grants in support of various aspects of this project.

A number of institutions have lent us materials, given permission for the use of photographs, provided access to records, sat for interviews, or shared valuable insights. The institutions, firms, and individuals that provided illustrations are acknowledged in the figure captions. We also want to thank individuals who helped us obtain the illustrations, including Annmarie Adams, Jennifer Bernatow, Barbara Bishop, Anna Christina Brattell, Eileen Callahan, Erica Collier, AlexAndréa DeLeón, Mary Ellen Devers, Ann Garrison, Steven Greenberg, Sarah Hartwell, Matt Jacques, Lorinda Klein, Mary McCann, Melissa Mileff, Teri Moffitt, Anne Ostendarp, Stacy Peeples, Erica Stoller, Anne Streeter, Kim Tenaglia, Katherine Watts, and Greg Williams. We want to thank the staff of Special Collections at the University of Southern California, especially Dace Taube in the Regional History Collection. Dace continues to provide a sanctuary for scholars. Peter Karpf, Mark Markiewicz, Nancy Shortsleeve, David Schwarz, and Suzanne Sullivan gave us interviews that were very valuable.

Diane Ghirado encouraged David to publish an early synopsis of the project in the *Journal of Architectural Education*. We wish to thank her for her support at a critical time in David's academic career. Dana Cook Grossman

XII

PREFACE AND ACKNOWLEDGMENTS

at *Dartmouth Medicine* published a version of the *JAE* article, which led us to several new sources of information. Paul Groth and Chris Wilson were instrumental in David's first presenting material on mini-mall medicine at a conference in memory of John Brinckerhoff Jackson, then publishing a version of it in their edited book. Alan Brandt coauthored a chapter on the evolution of the hospital with David in a book on the architecture of science, and he has been a loyal supporter of the project.

We want to thank the supportive people at Johns Hopkins University Press and the Center for American Places. George F. Thompson, president of the center, convinced us that not only could we write this book but that we should write it for this series. Randy Jones and others at the center saw us through many changes in the project. Through a long hiatus, the editors at Johns Hopkins University Press were very patient, especially Anne Whitmore, our expert and sympathetic copyeditor.

Lastly, we thank our family and friends. The Brookses, Conants, Crane-Chamberses, Karls, Boyntons, Sloanes, Steinbergs, and many others housed and fed us on research trips, talked to us about their experiences, guided us to important examples, and generally gave us aide and comfort. Drs. Steven Kairys, Jonathan Blitzer, and Carole Warde provided thoughtful comments on the healthcare system.

We appreciate the time and effort that all these people have put into making this book a reality. We also accept that any errors are completely our responsibility.

MEDICINE MOVES TO THE MALL

PROLOGUE: / The Evolving Architecture of Healthcare

Americans live in the age of the mall. The mall is no longer the rebel architectural entity it was in the 1950s, now claiming a spot in the retail landscape opposite its granddaddy, the department store, and its mother, the modern shopping center. It has matured and spawned mini-malls, superstores, and other new members of the retail clan. Today, the mall is influencing its surroundings, serving as a model for other types of developments, as a site for complex innovations, and even acting as the traditionalist confronted by upstarts such as entertainment retail complexes and the Internet. As religious scholar Ira Zepp asserts, shopping malls "have become so much a part of the everyday landscape that it is as hard to imagine an America without malls as it is to imagine an America without purple mountains and amber waves of grain."[1] Given the mall's success, why would it be surprising that even our most staid institutions, including the hospital and other healthcare facilities, have borrowed its design and have relocated their services into its storefronts?

Healthcare is ripe for new paradigms. Healthcare is changing, and changing fast. Although the federal government failed to institute a national health system in the early 1990s, the effort reflected a general recognition that the current American healthcare system is undergoing a rapid, largely undirected transformation. The rise of managed care organizations is one example. They barely existed a generation ago, now they are gobbling up every patient in sight. The crisis in healthcare insurance is another. Insurance is getting more expensive for many Americans and remains elusive for millions of others. Even the terms *doctor* and *patient* are being reconsidered. Alternatives ranging from *healthcare provider* and *client* to *medical professional* and *customer* have been suggested to replace the traditional labels. In simple terms, people believe that they used to know their healthcare provider better than they do today, that providers now read charts rather than know their patients, and that the practitioner does that chart reading between 15-minute clinical visits. The system costs over one trillion dollars, yet it seems less satisfactory with each passing day.

Healthcare is part of a whole world that is moving at a faster pace. Designers must create billboards that people can read while speeding by at 60 m.p.h. The developers of Universal Studio Hollywood's CityWalk speak seriously about the 5-square-mile "neighborhood" from which they draw patrons to their "street." Americans work harder and longer. They stay in touch by fax, e-mail, beeper, video conference, and cellular phone. A fan's cherished professional athlete will likely move on to a new team next year, and corporations seem less dedicated to their employees. Americans are constantly driving to the next obligation or adventure. In the many discussions that have accompanied the 2000 Census, society's mobility has drawn increasing attention from planners, architects, and social commentators who fear that people's transience diminishes their capability to maintain stable communities. Planning and design movements such as the "New Urbanism" and "Main Street America" call for a return to stability, intimacy, and neighborliness.

Transience in healthcare has become axiomatic. Every fall during open enrollment for employee benefits, people jump from one plan to another in search of a lower price or better quality, because they can no longer see the doctor as often as they would like or because payments for prescriptions are limited. Annually, physicians are dropped from one provider list and added to another. The relationship between doctor and patient—the most important element in healthcare—is less permanent. One visit, one doctor; another visit, another doctor, and the same with nurses, even receptionists. In a profession where not so long ago, practitioners congratulated themselves for their long, stable relationships with patients, transience has taken an enormous toll on doctors and patients. Many blame the government for meddling in healthcare. Others criticize insurers for setting rigid rules.

The transience arises from fundamental changes in medical practice as well as from insurance and governmental regulations. New anti-inflammatory drugs, anesthetics, pain medications, and antibiotics combine to make inpatient stays shorter or even unnecessary. Diseases such as pneumonia that in the recent past incapacitated people for weeks are typically handled on an outpatient basis. Even complex medical treatments are happening faster, with fewer days in the hospital. In 1995, the Johns Hopkins Oncology Center began performing some parts of bone marrow transplant procedures on an outpatient basis; instead of 45 days in the hospital, patients are in the center for 25 days, resulting in savings of $20,000 per patient. These savings are achieved by moving patients into a special outpatient residence, where a family member can aid in their recuperative care while providing a more homelike atmosphere for the patient.[2] In other words, shifting the location of care from the hospital to the hotel and the burden of care from the system to the patient's family.

A Changing Healthcare Landscape

The reinvention of the hospital, with its redesigned facilities, and the emergence of alternative sites for healthcare services, are the material for this study of the past, present, and future of the healthcare landscape in America. The word *landscape,* is used rather than *system* or *institution* because this study examines the place where medicine is practiced, not its organizational or economic structure. Cultural geographer Paul Groth has defined cultural landscape studies as those focusing "on the history of how people have used *everyday* space—buildings, rooms, streets, fields, or yards—to establish their identity, articulate their social relations, and derive cultural meaning."[3] This definition of *landscape* is not confined to pretty views or rural fields but can include places ranging from corporate campuses to the garage, as long as they are the spaces where everyday residents interact, play out their lives.

How has the place where medicine is performed changed over the last 150 years, and what is happening now? Specifically, how did the creation of the hospital represent not just a new way to practice medicine but also a new place to practice it? Then, how has the shopping mall, as well as other architectural models, influenced the new healthcare facilities that are being opened or redesigned today? Where is medical care performed, in what kind of building, with what kind of access to the public, and what kind of opportunities and obstacles for different genders, ethnicities, and income groups? All the answers to these questions are not clear. Indeed, the spatial relationship of patient to healthcare facility has received only fragmentary attention compared to the voluminous consideration of patients' financing of their healthcare or the shifting institutional relationship between physicians and patients. Can society ignore the places where healthcare is delivered and still understand the emerging system?

The new healthcare landscape contains virtually all the elements of past systems, but they are relocated, resituated, and reconfigured. The hospital is being redesigned to make it more accessible and familiar. Hospital managers are struggling to expand the hospital's relationship with patients as other forces work to "unbundle" hospital services. Procedures that have for the past century been migrating into the hospital are being relocated to sites that are more convenient to the public, easier for them to find, with a higher commercial profile. Americans' desire to know more about their health and their demand to be included in medical decisions have spawned a wide range of new programs to better inform them. The growth of the population needing long-term care has led to assisted living facilities and other types of care for elderly persons, along with significant changes in skilled nursing, just as the revolt against dying amid a roomful of machines has brought about the ever-expanding hospice movement.

Ironically, the success of modern biomedical research, often housed in the nation's hospitals, has encouraged the decentralization of medicine. Antibiotics have diminished the chances of postoperative infection, while new anesthetics make a patient's recovery from surgery much faster. Hospitals have become less necessary and hospital stays less common. Hospitals are closing because fewer beds are needed; patients no longer come as regularly or stay as long. As a result, patients never gain a sense of the place. Many ambulatory patients come repeatedly to the hospital but remain confused by its layout, intimidated by its design, and feel awkward and isolated even as they go into a building hoping for the exact opposite result.

These changes in healthcare practice have forced architects and hospital managers to search for models in places where Americans feel comfortable, where they can easily familiarize themselves. "To be understood," one prominent historian has written, "the hospital has to be seen . . . as an organ of society, sharing its characteristics, changing as the society of which it is a part is transformed, and carrying into the future evidence of its past."[4] Healthcare facilities reflect not only contemporary social characteristics but also physical ones. In the nineteenth century, the hospitals were civic or public enterprises whose designs mirrored the institution's moral mission. By early in the twentieth century, the modern hospital's façade symbolized society's faith in science and the hospital's mission as a functional place for curing disease.

Today, increasingly, hospitals and allied healthcare facilities share society's drive for convenience and service, diminishing the boundaries between sacred medicine and customer service. The concierge desk in the lobby of University of Southern California's University Hospital looks similar to the one in Nordstorm's department store at Los Angeles's Westside Pavilion shopping mall and like that in Pasadena's Ritz-Carlton Hotel. Such a change is an indication of a more comprehensive redesign of hospitals and healthcare facilities to evoke familiar spaces and expected services. The shopping mall and the hotel are not the only models from which designers have adapted characteristics to alter the relationship of the patient to the hospital's physical spaces. The home is also an important source. These three models, however, are particularly rich examples of that search, and the meaning of those changes for understanding the crisis in American healthcare.

An Evolving Landscape

Our exploration of the move of medicine to the mall revolves around three profound shifts. The first is the shift from the moral medicine that shaped the early American hospitals to the scientific medicine of the twentieth century. That shift was both shaped by new hospital designs and reinforced the new spatial relationships within those hospitals. Second was the contemporary critique and redesign of the spaces created for scientific medicine: the "postmodern" hospital deconstructed the rational scientific spatial configuration in favor of a more textured, accessible, and familiar place. Third, medical care is being decentralized through the relocation of services from the hospital to medical offices, many of which have moved to commercial venues. In the twenty-first century, care is increasingly likely to occur in a wide variety of settings as new antibiotics and anesthetics diminish the need to visit the hospital. As a result, the medical landscape as a whole, including healthcare facilities beyond the hospital, is being reconfigured to meet the new requirements of medical practice.

The story of the hospital is the tale of a public service transformed into a medical workshop. The evolution is an intricate account of the interweaving of technology, professionalism, and cultural attitudes. The American hospital began as a social benevolence harkening back to its European medieval ancestors and stylistically imitating its domestic contemporaries. It was established as an institution for the poor and for strangers. An institution that in the 1990s was a behemoth striding across the medical landscape, the hospital was hardly considered important as late as the 1870s. The horrors of the early hospitals were certainly exaggerated by advocates of their successor hospitals. However, when W. G. Wylie wrote in 1877 that "it would be a move in the wrong direction to offer an inducement to the sick, either poor or rich, to leave their homes and enter a hospital to be treated," he reflected the attitudes of many physicians and private citizens.[5] Even a generation later, far more Americans had never been admitted to a hospital than had.

By the middle of the twentieth century, new procedures greatly advanced surgical successes and innovative drug treatments increasingly served as defenses against a variety of debilitating diseases. Americans who had never visited a hospital found themselves going there for dramatic life-saving operations and increasingly for treatments of common illnesses. The hospital expanded, literally and figuratively. Patient floors, laboratories, and administrative functions were stacked on top of each other, or jumbled next to each other. Many small hospitals added building after building, tied together by mazes of hallways and marked by poorly placed directional signs. Either way, the hospital grew in prominence. Sometimes it sat, like a sacred temple, high on a hill over the town. Other times, it gobbled up neighborhoods as it stretched from building to building to building.

The successful rise of the hospital, though, was a Faustian bargain, as early commentators recognized. The modern hospital provided more technologically sophisticated treatments, a new standard of professionalism, a constantly expanding set of services, and a much better chance for survival. The package that these benefits came in was viewed with distaste. These spaces were often harsher, more sterile, and more mechanical than homes and doctors' offices. In 1918, architect William Ludlow asked whether hospitals had to have such an "austere aspect without" and "glaring white sterility within." Would they, he continued, always have to be "without cheer and without welcome"?

Even as machine medicine proliferated, the struggle to keep the hospital "homelike" continued. Ludlow, and commentators who followed him throughout the twentieth century, called for a "homelike hospital." Many hospitals began in renovated residences and only later were housed in larger buildings. In the twentieth century, wards were shrunk, to provide all patients with more privacy, as well as to rationalize the hospital as a work environment. The call for a caring place coexisted uneasily with the society's deep faith in medical science and biomedical technology, which would grow, not diminish, along with the centrality of the hospital in American healthcare.[6]

The notion that the hospital should be a home as well as a laboratory produced a growing ambivalence about the purpose of the institution. The many attempts to keep the hospital accessible, familiar and comfortable were secondary to the scientifically defined goal of curing illness and defeating death. Ultimately this hierarchy of priorities created an environment for change. In the 1960s, critics more forcefully asserted that the hospital seemed cold and distant, personnel more concerned with rules than with comfort. The entire system was faltering under its own reputation for saving lives and beating death. Americans had been led to believe that medicine could cure every disease, and then they found that it simply wasn't true. A crisis ensued, driven by changing economics, evolving practice, and people's growing skepticism.

The future of the hospital and the healthcare system is unclear given the current unstable circumstances. "A not insignificant number of the nation's fifty-three hundred or so acute-care hospitals are under siege," healthcare analyst Eli Ginzberg has written, "and . . . before the current period of turmoil comes to an end the hospital sector will be radically transformed as part of the broader transformation of the U.S. health-care system."[7] Will hospitals serve as comprehensive health centers with multifaceted services coexisting in the same space? Will they be the last resort of tertiary medicine, the home of the acutely ill? Whatever the configuration, two things seem to be certain: first, the hospital will continue to serve as the technological center of biomedical practice; second, hospital designs will be equally functional but more commercial than in past times. However, the balance between function and commerce, seriousness of purpose and accessibility are not yet settled, if they ever will be in this age of constant change.

The mall may seem an odd place to look for an alternative healthcare model. However, the mall (including the shopping center and the regional mall) and the mini-mall (also known as the micro-center, strip mall, commercial center, and several other possible phrases denoting similar streetside developments) have characteristics that soften the image of healthcare provision while increasing the convenience to patients and visitors. Architect H. Ralph Hawkins has written of healthcare malls: "The mall design offers an easily accessible, single complex that provides many healthcare services for the consumer, much like a neighborhood mall provides retail stores and amenities. . . . As a complex, the healthcare mall offers the typical consumer one-stop shopping that effectively meets a family's health needs."[8] Shopping malls are designed to direct people through space and encourage them to consume goods. The wayfinding devices embedded in mall designs are only rarely found in older hospitals, which all too often are a series of incrementally added spaces that rarely allow smooth circulation of pedestrian traffic. For instance, after several large additions, the UCLA Hospitals are notable for their lack of an obvious entrance. The university recently hired I. M. Pei to redesign the medical center and finally overcome this limitation. Examples of hospitals that are difficult to navigate abound in virtually every city. Unlike the physicians and hospital managers, who thought more about the needs of machines and the requirements of the regulators, mall developers understand that consumers need to have easy access, clear directions, and helpful signs along the way, or they won't come back to shop.

The characteristics of healthcare buildings play a role in shaping perceptions of healing, medical practice, and sickness itself. In the new generation of hospitals, ambulatory clinics, and specialty facilities, different messages are sent to patients, visitors, and staff than were sent by the previous generations of those buildings. The new hospital imports elements of the mall, hotel, and home as a means of altering the atmosphere and improving traffic circulation. Amid the new colors and textures, signs and posters, decorations and luxurious chairs, a new ethic of patient care is materializing. Patient-centered medicine empowers people to be involved in their care, to educate themselves about their illness, and to evaluate the people and the place that provide their care. That ethic has emerged slowly, because the forces of inertia are very strong, especially in terms of the physical requirements for a hospital. As health policy analyst Wanda Jones wrote in 1993, the "patient-focused concept is a powerful idea. . . . now we need a breakthrough for the hospital site itself."[9] No ideal model has been designed yet, but elements are now in hospitals scattered around the country.

The changing façade of medicine does not successfully remove continuing social inequities. The new medical malls provide the hospital with a new look, a more open and inviting appearance. Is everyone invited into this new hospital? Not always. The finances of health insurance continue to ordain a separate system of care for the poorest Americans and to offer a no-win choice for working-class families asked to decide between healthcare and other necessities. The deep financial divide drives the development of the medical mini-malls in cities' poorest neighborhoods as it shapes the decor in new hospitals attempting to attract patients in the wealthiest. This new healthcare landscape is tied inexorably to social issues. Historian George Rosen's claim that the hospital is "an organ of society" continues to be true.[10]

Mini-malls are more likely to be an object of derision than of study. Although the automobile culture that has shaped the development of the mini-mall is now more than a half-century old, architects, planners, historians, and urbanists continue to rail against them. New Urbanism, for instance, is an urban design and planning movement explicitly formed to combat the decentralization and perceived social isolation associated with car culture. As journalist James Howard Kunstler evocatively put it, "The new environment was designed primarily for the convenience of motorists, secondarily to assist corporations in moving vast volumes of merchandise via cars, tertiarily, for ease of maintenance, quatrarily for protection against lawsuits, and leastly, for the spiritual fulfillment of people. . . . The car-centered, car-*dominated*, human habitat can now be viewed—like Leninist economics—as an experiment that has failed."[11] Adherents of the New Urbanism reject the vernacular culture of the mini-mall, just as they abhor the cars that they believe have distorted the American way of life.

A "drive-in culture" of healthcare appears to be emerging.[12] Outpatient care has long occurred in places other than the hospital. Indeed, hospitals came late to this type of medical treatment. Before World War II, the doctor would visit people in their home, or they would go to the doctor's home. Today, while some people still go to the doctor's home with a clinic attached, most doctors have moved their practices away from their residence.

Many physicians have offices in the hospital itself, as staff of outpatient or ambulatory care clinics. Others have joined together and formed group practices that are situated in professional or medical office buildings. A growing number of these offices, though, are not located in separate medical offices with prestigious addresses, but in mini-mall clinics.

Mini-mall medicine responds to a multitude of issues confronting the healthcare system, including, critically, the disorganization that wastes so much of so many people's time. Healthcare management expert Regina Herzlinger has written that the healthcare system "is simply not organized to provide convenient care." Inconvenience may seem a trivial concern when compared to the weighty issues of life and death, but Herzlinger persuasively objects: "The . . . inconvenience of our healthcare system packs a deadly double punch. Not only does it rob people of their time, it prevents them from obtaining important preventive medical care."[13] Healthcare providers too easily ignore the obstacles that inconvenience aggravates; a mother's time constraints, a bus schedule, parking costs, work demands, all of which are exacerbated when someone has to wait, and wait, and wait to see the doctor. As Herzlinger reminds us, those hours could be spent making America more productive, taking care of families, earning a living, helping others, or socializing.

Not all mini-mall healthcare sites are equal. Even here the inequities embedded in American healthcare through the nation's history are very present. In poor neighborhoods clinics providing healthcare at inexpensive prices may also provide alternative medical treatments, or they may be under tremendous financial pressures or simply open and close unpredictably. And even though healthcare clinics are situated in commercial locations, they may still be open only to those who are insured or can pay cash for the services. The two-tiered system of healthcare does not disappear simply because physicians move outside the hospital; it is far more resilient than that.

However, establishing a University of California at San Francisco primary care clinic in a shopping center, for example, does alter the relationship of medicine and commerce, potentially producing a new relationship between patient and caregiver. These clinics are more accessible than any other healthcare location. Are they also dangerously close to lowering medical practice to the same level, in consumers' perception, as the stores that surround the clinics? Will patients perceive healthcare providers as having the same significance in their lives as shoe clerks? Are these clinics simply another place for the practice of medicine or a different place?

The redesign of the hospital and the establishment of medical mini-malls reflect a significant transformation of the healthcare system in America. Emerging out of the chaotic years associated with the introduction of fiscal competition within the American medical system, the new market-place of medical practice presages and reinforces the decentralization, com-mercialization, and demystification of medical practice. It raises real fears of franchise medicine, the incorporation of healthcare, even the specter of an oligarchy of medical companies. While these fears may be unfounded, the scientific hospital is no longer the black hole of medicine, attracting ever more procedures into its facility. Instead, market-driven medicine requires accessibility, convenience, and attractiveness. Rightly or wrongly, the issue of quality does not drive these developments anymore than it does the spread of HMOs and other managed care systems. Quality is an important concern. Whether the relocation of healthcare facilities into malls and mini-malls will improve quality, though, is something only the future can tell.

GALLERY ONE /   Machine Medicine

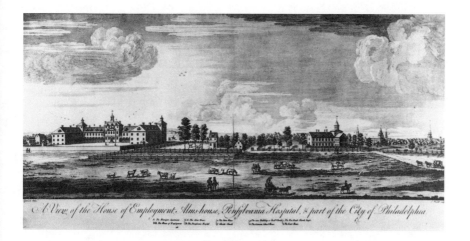

A View of the House of Employment, Alms-house, Pensylvania Hospital, & part of the City of Philadelphia

Philadelphia, circa 1755–60. The structure on the right is the earliest section of Pennsylvania Hospital, America's first general hospital, founded in 1755. Designed by Samuel Rhoads and Joseph Fox, it mirrored the large residences of the time, as did most buildings housing public charities, like the House of Employment, shown on the left. *Engraving by Hulet, courtesy of Pennsylvania Hospital Historic Collections, Philadelphia.*

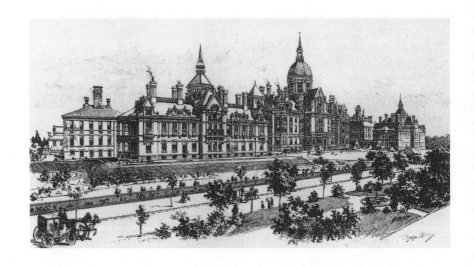

Baltimore, 1888. Johns Hopkins Hospital, designed by John Shaw Billings and John Niernsee and constructed between 1875 and 1885, established the pavilion plan as the standard for hospital design and introduced elaborate ventilation systems. *Wood engraving for Harper's Weekly, courtesy of the National Library of Medicine, Bethesda, Maryland.*

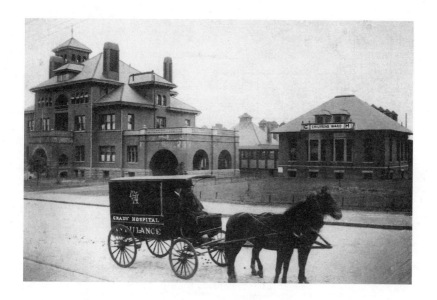

Atlanta, 1896. With the development of pediatrics as a medical specialty came a proliferation of hospitals or units devoted to the care of children, like the Children's Ward, at right, attached to Grady Hospital. Similar architectural differentiation followed the development of other specialities. *Photograph courtesy of the National Library of Medicine, Bethesda, Maryland.*

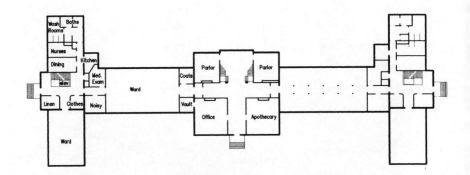

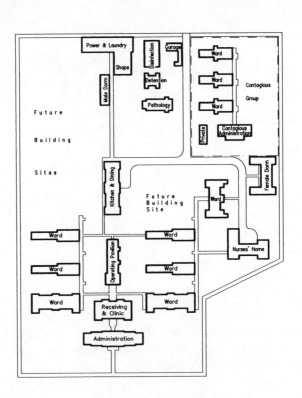

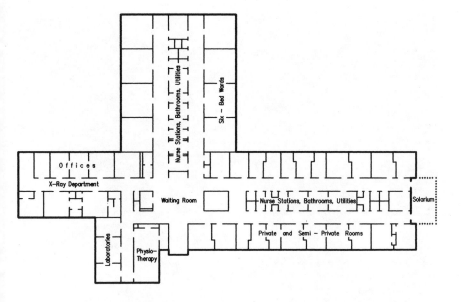

These three floor plans chronicle the evolution of hospital design. The 1755 plan by Samuel Rhoads and Joseph Fox for Pennsylvania Hospital (*above left*) followed the classic block style: central administrative building flanked by symmetrical wings. Samuel Hannaford and Sons' 1915 plan for Cincinnati General Hospital (*below left*) was a sprawling pavilion design in which hospital functions were clearly separated. Around 1947 Charles F. Neergaard produced an updated "double pavilion" plan (*above*) that placed the services in a central core, shortened the patient corridors, and gave each patient room more light and air. *Adapted from* Report of the Board of Managers of the Pennsylvania Hospital, *Philadelphia, 1897; Edward F. Stevens,* The American Hospital of the Twentieth Century, *1928; and Isadore Rosenfield,* Hospitals: Integrated Design, *1947.*

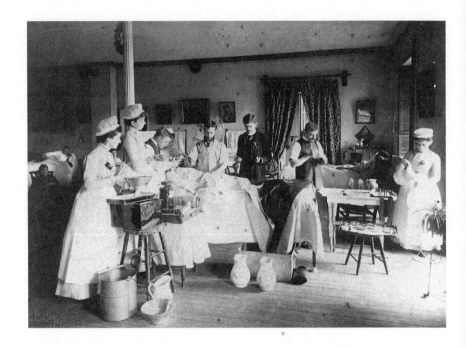

New York City, circa 1891. Bellevue Hospital had two operating rooms at this time, but for whatever reason the operation captured in this photograph was being performed on the ward, with other patients looking on. While the curtains and plant indicate the domestic feel of hospital wards, the use of surgical gloves and anesthesia represent advances in medical science. *Photograph by Oscar Gelason Mason, courtesy of the Bellevue Hospital Center Archives, Board of Managers Collection.*

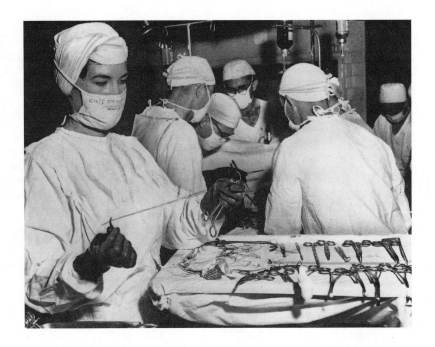

Los Angeles, circa 1959. In the hospital as medical workshop, the patient has virtually disappeared from sight, as the focus is on the specific organ or physiological manifestation of disease. Machinery dominates this operating room in White Memorial Hospital. *Courtesy of the University of Southern California, on behalf of the USC Library Department of Special Collections.*

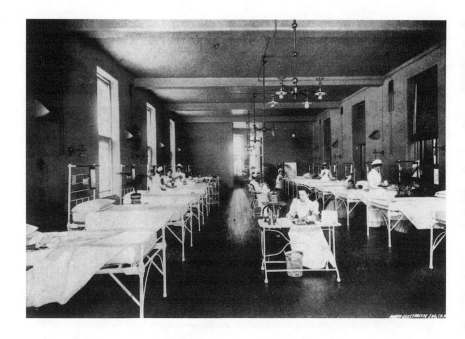

Cincinnati, 1940s. Large open wards defined both the earliest and the pavilion-style hospitals. Populated mostly by the "worthy poor," they were easily supervised but not private. In some hospitals, the patients and staff attempted to make them more homelike. In others, like this 24-bed ward in Cincinnati General Hospital, they were stark reminders that their occupants were in need of charity. *Courtesy of the National Library of Medicine, Bethesda, Maryland.*

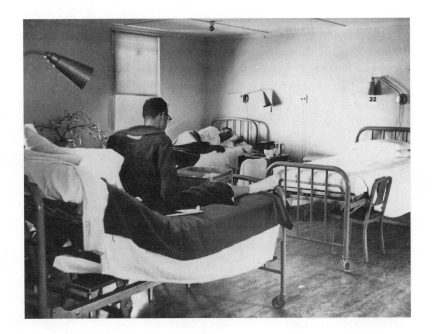

Long Beach, California, 1960. The large ward as the norm gradually gave way to smaller ones, like this four-bed ward at Long Beach General Hospital. Semiprivate rooms with modern conveniences, such as a private telephone line and a television, eventually replaced the ward, even in many public hospitals. *Courtesy of the University of Southern California, on behalf of the USC Library Department of Special Collections.*

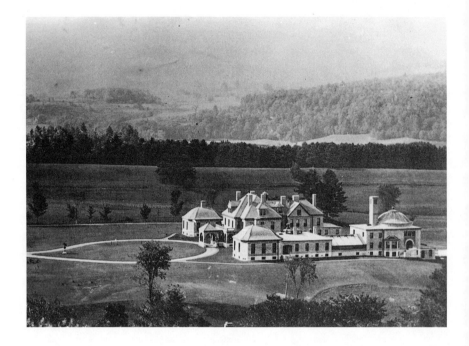

Hanover, New Hampshire, 1892 and 1952. Expansion of hospitals created some architectural oddities. Faulkner House (*facing page*), designed by Ellerbee and Company, was situated directly in front of Mary Hitchcock Memorial Hospital (*above*), the original building of which had been designed by Rand and Taylor but which had been growing outward for 60 years. Such expansions created pedestrian mazes. At Mary Hitchcock, people followed colored tapes on the floor to navigate their way through the complex of buildings. *Photographs courtesy of the Dartmouth College Library.*

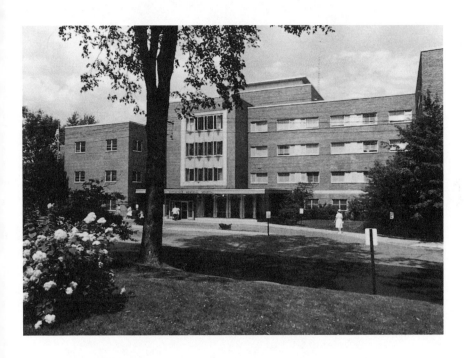

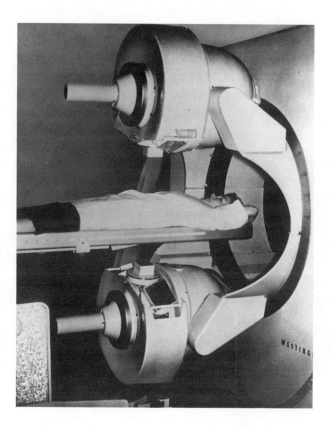

Duarte, California, 1958. Science and technology are important foundations of modern medicine. Here, the cesium ring, firing "hot atoms," is used in cancer treatment for the first time in the United States, at City of Hope Hospital in a suburb of Los Angeles. New technologies offered hope to desperate patients. They also consumed larger and larger spaces, forcing hospitals to expand repeatedly in buildings that were rarely designed for such flexibility. *Courtesy of the University of Southern California, on behalf of the USC Library Department of Special Collections.*

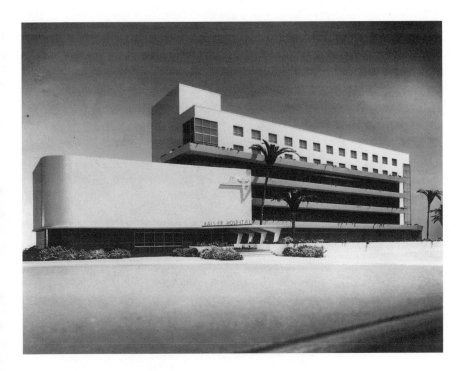

Los Angeles, 1953. The sleek modernist design of Kaiser Foundation Medical Center, created by Wolf and Phillips, architects noted for hospital design, was stripped of earlier civic and moralistic sensibilities and reflected instead the functionalism, rationalism, and scientific orientation of clinical medicine at mid-century. *Photograph of architect's model courtesy of the University of Southern California, on behalf of the USC Library Department of Special Collections.*

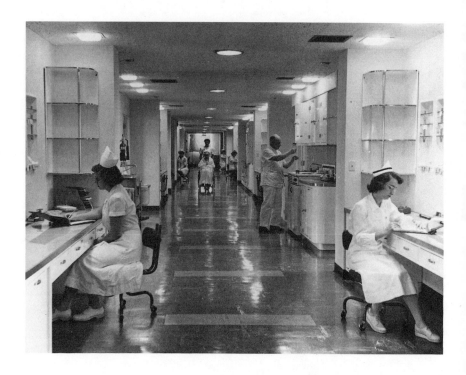

Los Angeles, 1953. Inside the 7-story, 224-bed Kaiser Foundation Medical Center, designed by Wolf and Phillips, separating public corridors from staff corridors shielded visitors from some of the tragic sights associated with hospital care. The decentralized nursing stations were intended to improve efficiency. *Courtesy of the University of Southern California, on behalf of the USC Library Department of Special Collections.*

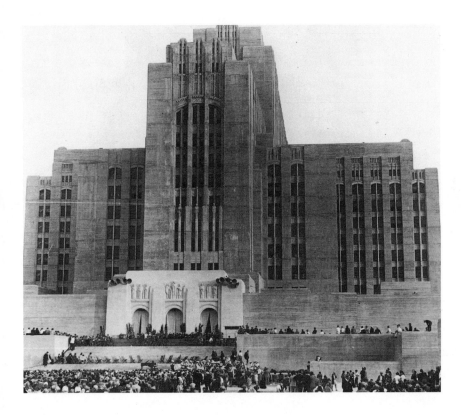

Los Angeles, 1933. The monolithic Los Angeles County General Hospital, designed by Allied Architects, symbolized the emergence of the hospital as a citadel of healthcare, a medical skyscraper. *Courtesy of the University of Southern California, on behalf of the USC Library Department of Special Collections.*

ONE / The Medical Workshop

I n the middle of the Great Depression, several thousand people gathered to dedicate the new Los Angeles County Hospital. The 20-story unpainted concrete building was huge on any scale. Housing 2,444 patient beds (3,600 in an emergency), sophisticated laboratories, and extensive teaching facilities, the new hospital epitomized the modern hospital's diverse institutional mission.[1] It towered over neighboring buildings. Its central hallways were the lengths of football fields, planned to have five or six 24-bed wards per floor. Its patient and staff census equaled the population of a small city. Later the hospital would be formally renamed the Los Angeles County–University of Southern California (LAC-USC) Medical Center, signifying the close relationship between the medical school's education, training, and research activities with the clinical care occurring in the hospital's wards.

County Hospital was representative of the remarkable change and continuity one finds in the history of the American hospital. As late as 1870, no one could have imagined that by the 1930s Americans of all incomes would have embraced the hospital as a site for their health care. However, not only were thousands of new hospitals established between 1870 and 1930, but existing ones were constantly expanding. Sometimes, older buildings were replaced with new ones, as at County. Other times, new construction enlarged existing structures or expanded them. All the new spaces were necessary to accommodate the constantly expanding arsenal of medical technology. Los Angeles County Hospital, like hospitals around the country, was filled with new and exciting medical innovations. Its corridors were populated by doctors and nurses, laboratory technicians, and a variety of technical support personnel who were educated in new clinically based education sequences that had, in the minds of contemporaries, dramatically improved the standard of care.

At the same time, Los Angeles County Hospital was part of an almost two-century-long tradition of hospital care for the least fortunate Americans. This public charity continued to serve the county's poor even amid an array of high technology and highly trained staff. Although in the twentieth century smaller wards replaced the large wards of the eighteenth, they were still spaces where privacy was a secondary concern. The medical staff controlled admissions (doctors having wrested control from civilian overseers a generation or two earlier), but in either hospital, patients relinquished control to the institution's guardians. New medicines, surgical techniques, and other advances resulted in much higher rates of recovery for twentieth-century patients, but medicine still struggled with many mysteries.

The emergence of the modern hospital was an evolution, not a revolution. Three stages of development occurred over the course of the maturation of hospital architecture, and often within the life span of an individual hospital. America's first general hospital, as well as most initial buildings of the hospitals that followed during the next 150 years, was a renovated house. The house provided an economical starting point for a hospital association just starting out. Before the twentieth century, the home was the primary place for medical care for everyone in society, so the hospitals used an institutional setting that imitated the preferred and common one. Later, the first buildings constructed as hospitals continued this relationship, being designed to draw comparison with the grand domestic residences of the day.

During the second evolutionary stage, even before modern medicine embraced the germ theory, the shifting ideas about disease transmission produced the first unique hospital building style, the pavilion. The pavilion design allowed patients to be separated from one another at a time when hospital death rates from contagion and infection continued to be very high. The pavilion also signaled the victory of the physician over the trustee, and the shift in the hospital's mission from moral education to clinical therapy. In the third stage, which occurred during most of the twentieth century, hospitals built upward and housed medicine's specialists and their marvelous machines. The modern hospital retained elements of the older one but accumulated new services that demanded different spaces and redirected organization. Designers and managers struggled to balance the dual roles of the hospital as scientific laboratory and patient's home away from home.

The story of medicine's modern transformation from those earliest hospitals to the modern behemoths like LAC-USC has been well told by medical historians. However, the buildings have typically been treated only as backdrops in those stories, depicted as passive receptacles in which the heroic deeds of physician scientists produced innovations in medicine. The buildings' architects and managers were active participants in the changes associated with modern medicine. Their designs not only reflected innovations in medical practice but codified and validated them; they even at times anticipated them. The hospital came to symbolize an emergent healthcare system in which a new style of medicine was practiced. Patients were enticed out of their homes into specialized spaces housing innovative technology; the hospital offered patients services that were impossible to undertake in a domestic environment. The result was that physicians and medicine gained a new prestige that reinforced the centrality of the hospital in the healthcare system.

Home-Style Medicine

Americans living before the Civil War would not understand the modern hospital's centrality in the healthcare system. They believed that illness was inextricably tied to a person's familial history, physical constitution, and social environment. A disease did not commence upon the transmission of specific bacteria or viruses, but because of a patient's predisposition through heredity or moral standing and because of changes in the weather, the use of alcohol, or a sudden heightened anxiety. The disease could have started in the womb, if the mother was too excitable, or even before if the father had drunk wine before intercourse. Since the factors were so complicated, and interrelated, diagnosis was both problematic and tentative. A blow to the head was easily understood, the sudden onset of cholera in an upstanding merchant's daughter considerably less so. The moral standing of a person—their social standing, economic success or failure, religious beliefs, etc.—influenced both how their illness was diagnosed and the treatment prescribed.

The physician's role was as much social as curative. Physicians lacked the necessary tools to resolve illness. They relied instead on social and environmental explanations for the onset of disease. The better a physician knew the patient, and the patient's family and ancestors, the better the diagnosis. As historian Morris Vogel has written, "ideally, [the doctor] offered advice and treatment appropriate for the contexts within which the patient lived and worked."[2] By knowing a patient's heredity, home life, work habits—a person's strengths and weaknesses—the physician would better understand possible "causes" of disease and limits of treatments.

The parlor and the bedroom were the usual places for medical visits and interventions. Physicians were called to the home to oversee the progress of an illness and might visit several times a day, day after day, for weeks. Up to early in the nineteenth century, "heroic" therapeutic measures would have been used, primarily bloodletting and such emetics as calomel. When George Washington developed his mortal respiratory illness in December 1799, three physicians came to Mount Vernon. They blistered and bled him to no avail.[3] By mid-century, physicians had become more conservative, assuming that diseases were "self-limited," that they had a typical life span. If left alone, the tendency of human health would be toward life not death, so measures that debilitated the patient might change the natural course of the disease. Surgery, as dangerous as it was, would be employed in obvious cases of injuries or desperate conditions of infection and tumors. Otherwise, the care consisted of watching, waiting, and applying a small assortment of medicines.

Middle-class Americans viewed the decision to remove the patient from the home as disastrous, since only in the home could the physician appropriately understand the patient and the environmental influences upon his or her health. Only there could the natural balances that were the goal of contemporary therapies be achieved, through careful examination of family relations, diet, and domestic surroundings. Further, why remove a patient? The therapeutic procedures available to physicians before the mid-nineteenth century were achievable in the home. Diagnosis, treatment, even surgery could be conducted there. Besides, few alternatives to treatment at home were available.

Home as Hospital

Receiving care at home presumed a network of family caregivers and the means to pay the visiting physician. Those who did not have either had to rely on an unsystematic assemblage of public care. The alternatives included physicians' charity, outpatient dispensaries (almost exclusively in large cities), and institutional care. The last of these options ranged from the unreliable medical care available in the poorhouses and almshouses to, for those who were morally acceptable and suffering from only certain diseases, a small number of general hospitals. The comparative rates of survival in these alternative sites are unknown; however, none was an ideal choice.

The first American general hospital was founded at Philadelphia in 1751 at the urging of, among others, Benjamin Franklin. The original Pennsylvania Hospital was in John Kinsey's home, refurbished for this purpose. This rough wooden structure served only a few years, until a new hospital building could be constructed. However, it was representative of many generations of hospitals in the United States. For instance, in southern California, virtually all the current major hospitals can trace their origins to residences. San Diego's St. Joseph's Sanitarium and Hospital started out in two rented rooms above a men's clothing store, while the Los Angeles Infirmary (later St. Vincent's Hospital) was housed in the former adobe residence of Don Cristobal Aguilar, one of the area's early rancheros. Kaspar Cohn, the first Jewish hospital in Los Angeles and the predecessor to the prestigious Cedars-Sinai Medical Center, opened in a Victorian gingerbread house. Los Angeles's Children's Hospital was established in 1901 in a small home near downtown, and Orthopaedic Hospital opened in 1922 in the refurbished stables of an old estate. These southern California hospitals were typical of initial efforts in towns and cities nationwide. Most institutions had to slowly accumulate support before constructing substantial buildings.

In many smaller towns and suburbs, the original home hospital survived well into the twentieth century. As late as 1921, Edward F. Stevens, then the leading hospital architect in North America, described redesigning a residential house into a hospital in his widely read book on hospital architecture.[4] He described how the old Choate house in Woburn, Massachusetts, had been quite easily adapted in 1909 into a hospital of "moderate proportions." The grand parlor made an "excellent five-bed ward . . . , while the sitting room served as a children's ward, and the little den as the hospital office." In a sentence that must amaze and amuse present-day designers, he noted that the kitchen and laundry were sufficient as they were for the needs of the hospital. In 1916, the rapidly changing needs of medicine forced that hospital's managers to ask Stevens to improve the building, since they needed a surgical facility, more private rooms, and a maternity department.

THE MEDICAL WORKSHOP

With a compatible addition to the original facility, Stevens easily doubled the hospital's capacity from 14 to 33 and provided two operating rooms, an ambulance entrance, and other space for laboratories and x-ray machines. The improved hospital retained the look of a manor house but was outfitted to accommodate modern medical diagnosis and treatment.

The initiation of hospitals in residences was obviously primarily for fiscal reasons. Few hospital associations could afford to construct a major building immediately upon formation. Few were lucky enough to have a benefactor prepared to underwrite such a venture. Instead, they opened in an adapted home, then only later moved into a specially designed building. However, the home was more than a convenience. Home hospitals were intended to be welcoming and reassuring to patients who feared institutional care. Even after early hospital founders acquired sufficient funds to build a separate facility, they continued to rely on the residence as their design model.

Hospital as Home

In 1756, Pennsylvania Hospital opened the first wing of its new facility, a more majestic, Federal-style building designed by Samuel Rhoads and Joseph Fox. The new building had roughly the same floor plan as the Edinburgh Royal Infirmary (opened in 1738), a decision perhaps influenced by the Edinburgh education of Dr. Thomas Bond, another of the original promoters of the hospital. The three-story hospital was designed to have two patient wings extending from a central building, forming an H. Construction ultimately took more than 50 years, with the east patient wing (1756) and west patient wing (1796) opening before the joining portion (1804). When the central building finally opened, it became the grand domestic center of the facility. It was taller and more imposing than the wings, because it was raised one story above them. In addition, its roof extended over the wings sufficiently to cover their cornices. The central building held apartments for the staff, a dining room, kitchen, parlor, and library, as well as the administrative offices and America's first hospital-based pharmacy. Wards for male patients were on the first floor, those for women on the second. Mentally ill patients were housed in the basement. The wings also held a small number of private rooms for paying patients. Rooms for these patients' servants were in the attics, above which on each wing was a cupola, which provided additional ventilation for the wards. The hospital's setting was bucolic, according to contemporary engravings and descriptions. As late as the beginnings of the Revolution, the hospital was outside the built-up portions of the city, set in a square bounded by 8th Street, 9th Street, Spruce, and Pine.[5]

The Pennsylvania Hospital's design was far from revolutionary. Indeed, in a late 1750s engraving of the House of Employment and Pennsylvania Hospital, the structures resemble each other. The House of Employment is the most complete, with its central block, lateral sections, and large terminal wings. The Alms-House is a much smaller homelike building surrounded by outbuildings. At the time of the engraving, the hospital consisted of only the east wing with its cupola. Although the three institutions had different and distinguishable missions, the structures suggested that they were designed to embody contemporary domestic values, through identification with the grand domestic structures of the time, and to provide "inmates" a morally appropriate and instructive environment.

Pennsylvania Hospital and the hospitals that slowly opened in cities and towns around the nation were intended to serve only those "worthy poor" who were not suffering from contagious or morally unacceptable diseases. These new institutions, such as New York Hospital and Massachusetts General Hospital, were intended to allow working people of integrity who could not afford "decent" home medical treatment to receive it without suffering the indignities of mingling with the morally corrupt, as the occupants of almshouses and poorhouses were presumed to be. The new hospitals were staffed primarily by physicians offering their services for no fee, establishing a relationship between physician and institution that still exists in most American "voluntary" hospitals, nonprofit charitable organizations. The new hospitals were instruments of society not medicine, managed by boards of lay trustees not physicians, part of the extensive network of social charities noted by Alexis de Tocqueville in *Democracy in America* (1835–40).

As late as 1873, a survey of hospitals reported only 178 nationwide, 128 of which were general hospitals. These general hospitals served the urban poor almost exclusively, as either public services or private charities.[6] Just as Europe's eighteenth-century hospital movement rose largely from urban growth, America's first hospitals were in the nation's largest cities, where the poor lived in the greatest numbers, and strangers, far from the comforts of their own homes, were in the greatest need of help when they suffered sickness. These two groups represented economic disparity and social disorder to the benefactors and managers who shaped the early hospitals. In an institution so fundamentally associated with the disorder of disease—the uncontrolled aspects of disability, suffering, and death—order and control became paramount values in its organization and design.

Lay hospital trustees were responsible for the hospitals' construction and operation. They constantly felt a need to justify the new institutions. The grand façades that adorned most early hospitals reflected this need to reassure the public of the hospital's purpose and role in society. They were not an escape from responsibility, nor a refuge for the immoral. Instead, they were civic institutions, public charities, necessary in a civilized society. Hospitals were places of propriety and moral purpose. Their design reflected this social mission rather than any specific notion of the nature of disease, its transmission, or medical practice. Medicine remained subordinate to the moral ideals of the benefactors.

To gain entrance to the new hospitals, patients usually had to provide a reference from a social accepted person testifying to their good character. After being admitted, their social standing might affect their fees and care. At the Infants' Hospital in New York in the 1860s, the charge was $7 a month for ambulatory services; if the child was illegitimate, the fee was $10. Patients were often expelled if they violated the hospital's rigid rules, which forbade rude language and card playing while demanding that most convalescent patients work, nursing other, sicker patients and maintaining the facility. Visiting was severely limited, sometimes to one visitor a day for no more than one hour, and none on Sundays. Except, of course, for the lay trustees, who could patrol the wards at any time to ensure their moral atmosphere.

The early hospitals each had a central structure from which the wards extended. These central buildings served as the administrative headquarters of the new institutions. They provided offices for the overseers, matrons, clerks, and other administrative staff. At Pennsylvania and New York hospitals, a pharmacy was integrated into the first floor plans. Passing through the grand façade, visitors often entered a parlor. Such amenities suggested the elegant residences that the administrative buildings were intended to replicate. The hospital was the practical and symbolic equivalent of a home away from home. Since patients were being morally as well as physically healed, the domestic environment was a crucial design feature.

The wards were large and divided by gender and financial arrangement. When the new Massachusetts General Hospital opened in 1821, the wards held approximately 20 beds in square rooms with stoves in the middle. New York physician John Jones hoped to convince New York Hospital administrators to limit wards to a maximum of 8 patients, but in reality the number was doubled. Beds were typically lined up against the outer wall, facing inward to the fireplace or stove that warmed the ward. Some wards had small tables next to the beds, but in general the furnishings were very sparse and economical. Curtains shielded the top of the bed, and thus the patient's head, from the view of the patient on either side, but privacy was almost nonexistent.

A small staff of nurses easily supervised the large wards. Patients had little control over their environment. In 1876, John Shaw Billings, wrote of the existing urban hospitals:

> To be an "inmate" was to barter independence for security, to subject oneself to the physical and moral authority of trustees, administrators, and attending physicians. . . . [Patients] are placed in a large, bright room, with perhaps twenty others; on one side may be a man dying, on the other a blackguard conversing with a visitor of like stamp. Every movement is under observation, and to many persons this is very unpleasant.[7]

Additionally, their day was carefully routinized. Their feedings, tasks, and communication with the outside world were tightly scheduled. Trustees and physicians did not always agree over the primary purpose of the hospital. Physicians increasingly viewed hospitals as clinical training grounds, while trustees continued to view them as social benefits. John Green, in his 1861 book on city hospitals, summarized the issue when he wrote, "Hospitals are essentially charitable institutions, and the welfare of the patient must ever hold the first place in the minds of their founders. Nevertheless, we must not lose sight of the fact, that they are also our great schools of clinical observation and instruction; and have thus, perhaps, rendered their most important service to mankind."[8] The Philadelphia Board of Guardians of the Poor saw it differently, as they stated in 1845: "There are rights possessed even by the recipients of charity, which should be guarded, and feelings which should be respected."[9] They feared particularly that young male medical students' examination of female patients and postmortem examinations might excite the community against their institutions. Ultimately, perhaps, they feared that the priorities of the physicians would gain ascendancy over their focus on moral order. If they did worry about the latter, they were right to do so. The hospital of the early twentieth century would have an emphasis on discipline no less rigid than that of earlier hospitals, but morality would be replaced by science.

The Great Expansion

In 1877, a physician named W. Gill Wylie wrote, "Civilization has not reached that state of perfection in which hospitals can be dispensed with." Wylie's pessimistic prediction reflected his belief that the hospital was a necessity, but only for the poor and homeless, those stranded from their families, in the armed services, or the insane. Wylie had concluded, after studying mortality at Bellevue Hospital in New York City, "The truth is, the majority of our hospitals . . . are liable to do more harm than good." He protested the trend of a small but growing number of middle-class and wealthy Americans using hospitals. "Now, it seems to us that it would be a move in the wrong direction to offer an inducement to the sick, either poor or rich, to leave their homes and enter a hospital to be treated." The home, not the hospital, was the appropriate place for medical care, in the opinion of physicians. The hospital was an institution of last resort, primarily for those who had no other alternatives.[10]

Roughly forty years later, a surgeon named Robert Morris could look back over his fifty years of practice and reflect on the public's changed attitude toward hospitals. "Dread of them was general and well founded before the days of antiseptic surgery. But with its widespread adoption, fear faded rapidly from the lay mind." While Morris was overly optimistic in his assessment of how rapidly and completely the public had embraced the hospital, he rightly noted the hospital's remarkable transformation in the public's mind. As Morris continued, "few people would go voluntarily" to the hospital in the old days, but by 1930 he could say, "almost everybody with any illness at all serious wishes to go there."[11] The new, improved hospital had become a general benefit.

As a result, the number of hospitals grew dramatically. As late as the 1820s, the United States had three general hospitals, Pennsylvania, New York, and Massahcusetts General. The 1873 study found 138 general hospitals. By 1904, the United States boasted over 1,493 hospitals. Those hospitals admitted over one million patients, who stayed an average of 25 days.[12] A healthcare system had been born. Community and proprietary hospitals in small towns joined prestigious metropolitan academic hospitals in large cities. Some hospitals were open to all, others limited to ethnic, religious, or other communities. Some hospitals treated all types of conditions, others focused on special patient populations, like children and pregnant women. Together they represented the foundation of the twentieth-century healthcare system.

From an architectural perspective, the expansion had two stages. Starting after the Civil War, the urbanizing and industrializing nation needed to respond to a growing population that could no longer depend on family or social networks for their healthcare. So, in the first stage, starting in the 1870s, the United States embraced the pavilion-style hospital, a building form developed expressly to respond to medical concerns about transmission of disease. In these pavilions, physicians and nurses initiated a series of medical innovations that would dramatically improve patient outcomes and bolster public impressions of the hospital. The success of these pavilion hospitals spawned new generations of hospitals in large and small cities alike.

A second stage started in the 1920s, when rich, poor, and middle class began accepting the hospital as a medical necessity. While the pavilion model was still influencing hospital architecture three generations after its introduction, the modern "vertical hospital," with its more efficient use of land, began appearing. The vertical hospital has remained the primary form of the hospital until very recently, even though its external appearance and internal arrangements have adapted to changes in architectural fashions and medical practice. Stylistic shifts would mirror a substantive institutional redirection of the hospital from moral charity to medical workshop driven by the rationalism of modern science.

THE MEDICAL WORKSHOP

The move from a moral to a scientific hospital did not occur miraculously with the coming of the new century. The hospital underwent a slow evolution that was belied by the sudden coalescence of the institution in the first decades of the twentieth century. A critical first step toward the modern hospital was taken when hospital architects offered a particular design for the hospital. The pavilion-plan hospital represented a significant step in separating the hospital from other charitable institutions and in establishing a medical rationale for the hospital's form. The new design did not mimic other buildings but was purposefully constructed to serve as a medical facility. As architectural historian Christine Stevenson notes of the pavilion-style hospital, "It looks liked nothing else: . . . the building type abandoned its ecclesiastical, monastic, and domestic antecedents."[13] Instead, the new hospital embodied contemporary theories of disease transmission and medical treatment, subtly altering the power relationship between physician and trustee.

In mid-nineteenth-century America, medicine had few answers for the contagious and infectious diseases that ravaged the nation's cities and towns. Europeans and Americans, who were increasingly unwilling to accept that disease was a divine retribution, were still unable to prove the existence of specific causes for diseases. Physicians could not even agree how such diseases were transmitted, but many feared it was through a "miasma." The concept of the miasma has a long history, dating back to the Greeks. "The exact nature or character of these miasmas remained undefined," as historian Caroline Hannaway has written. The "general sources of the putrefaction of the air included stagnant marshes and pools, vapours from a variety of sources including corpses of humans and animals, sick persons, excreta, spoiled foodstuffs, decaying vegetable matter, and exhalations that came from the ground through rupture or clefts." Fears of miasma motivated many social reform and public health activities during the nineteenth century, including battles against overcrowded housing conditions, the relocation of garbage dumps and cemeteries, and a host of other struggles to clean the air and land of the city.[14]

These fears of miasma were reinforced by the high death tolls of contagious and infectious diseases. High rates of urbanization in the late eighteenth and early nineteenth centuries overwhelmed cities, which were unprepared for the onrush of migrants and immigrants they experienced. As one of the nation's leading proponents of public health measures sarcastically reported in 1850, "London, with its imperfect supply of water,—its narrow crowded streets,—its foul cesspools,—its hopeless pauperism,—its crowded graveyards, and its other monstrous sanitary evils, is as healthy a city as Boston, and in some respects more so."[15] Infectious diseases, such as yellow fever, raged periodically. Cholera appeared suddenly in 1832 and returned with terrifying incidence again in 1849 and 1866. Influenza and pneumonia were almost always present, along with a growing number of cases of tuberculosis, diphtheria, scarlet fever, and measles. Until near the end of the century, most medical people believed that such diseases were at least encouraged by miasmas, if not directly transmitted through them.

Even though hospital trustees barred contagious patients from admittance, the hospital was perceived to be a place where one was likely to contract diseases. "Hospitalism"—the transmission of diseases in hospitals—reinforced persistent public concerns about the danger of hospitals. Old-style hospital buildings, especially the large common wards, were perceived to be home to miasma, since they housed a mass of decomposing or putrid flesh. "When a ward is overcrowded, or the ventilation insufficient," architect John Woodworth noted in 1876, "the miasma generated by the patients accumulates, permeating the walls and ceilings, pervading the clothing and bedding, lodging in the cracks of the floor and on the furniture." As a result, the ward became "a propagating house of erysipelas, gangrene, puerperal fever, and other preventable diseases."[16] Everywhere in the ward was a possible hiding place for potentially dangerous materials. The only hopes were isolation, ventilation, and cleanliness. Just as public health sanitarians were cleaning the cities, hospital designers and managers tried ensuring the healthiness of the wards.

Florence Nightingale was so concerned about the dangers of hospitals that she proclaimed:

> It may seem a strange principle to enunciate as the very first requirement in a hospital that it should do the sick no harm. It is quite necessary nevertheless to lay down such a principle, because the actual mortality in hospitals . . . is very much higher than any calculation founded upon the mortality of the same class of patient treated out of hospital would make one expect.[17]

THE MEDICAL WORKSHOP

Such fears led several physicians and architects to propose razing hospitals on a regular basis, perhaps every fifty years, to avoid the effects of the accumulation of miasmic contaminants. Others sought to build hospitals that were so well ventilated that the contaminants could be controlled. Their search for a safely ventilated hospital resulted in the worldwide acceptance of the pavilion as the building's key design component.

The pavilion originated as an ornamental building for the very rich. Most famous were the pavilion pleasure houses of Louis XIV at Marly (1695), his retreat from the more majestic and formal Versailles. The style was gradually adapted to other uses by European architects. The French experimented with it for hospital design in the post-Revolutionary era, and European architectural and medical communities embraced it starting in the mid-nineteenth century.[18] The pavilion was widely adopted as the model for hospitals partly because Florence Nightingale's name became associated with a popular pavilion ward design. Nightingale's Crimean War experience convinced her of the need for greater space between patients, better air flow through wards, the healthy influence of light, and the need for isolation of various diseases from each other (especially separate wards' ventilation systems). Air, space, light, and isolation were deemed important because they defeated the miasma, by dissipating its effects and controlling its origins. Nightingale calculated precise recommendations for the distribution and allocation of space inside the hospital, suggesting 1,500 cubic feet per patient, 100 square feet for each bed. Each ward was to be situated in its own narrow, one- or two-story pavilion with high ceilings allowing greater control over ventilation as well as defeating any chances of disease transmission.[19]

Americans used a version of the pavilion plan for battlefield hospitals during the Civil War but only truly accepted the form after the publicity surrounding the construction of Johns Hopkins Hospital. Johns Hopkins, begun in 1875 and opened in 1885, was America's exemplar of the pavilion-plan hospital. In 1907, surgeon A. J. Oschner could reflect that "It was . . . the work which was done by the commission in charge of the construction of the Johns Hopkins Hospital which attracted the greatest amount of attention everywhere and which virtually popularized the low pavilion plan."[20] The hospital's trustees asked four leading physicians to propose alternative designs, then they printed the plans in a widely influential compilation. After the long, inconclusive design competition, the trustees worked with

John Shaw Billings, their consultant and former surgeon general of the United States, and John Niernsee, their executive architect, to develop plans for the hospital. The design surrounded the buildings with light, air, and sun, while separating patients by illness. The wards had elaborate ventilation systems that ensured that contaminated air would be quickly and effectively removed before it harmed another patient. Johns Hopkins received a great deal of contemporary attention, and from then on the pavilion plan was used throughout the country.

The Hopkins plan was resolutely symmetrical. The administration building stood at the center of the design, with the apothecary directly behind it. Flanking it were female and male "pay-wards," the kitchen, and the nurses' home. Offset and extending out in a long row behind the administration building were the common wards. Four rectangular wards and one octagonal ward had been constructed behind the female pay-ward when the hospital opened in 1885. The octagonal ward was an experiment to test competing techniques of ventilation. The hospital's architectural plan called for a similar long row to be built behind the male pay-ward, but the hospital eventually used this land for other purposes. Each building was reached through a corridor, and each was isolated from the others by these corridors. The laundry and pathology buildings were also symmetrically located in relationship to the administration building. The dispensary and surgical amphitheater were the only buildings with no intended counterpart.

While discussions of Johns Hopkins Hospital often began with its decorative glories, which reflected the hospital's continuing civic presence, the remaining description typically focused on the wonders of its construction, especially the new ventilation systems in the common wards. A physician, Christian Holmes, surveying hospital construction in 1911, asserted that each Hopkins ward was "a small, but complete hospital."[21] The pavilion plan heightened this sense of completeness. The trustees of Johns Hopkins considered ventilation so important that they experimented with two different systems of airflow within the individual wards. They also tried out three different ward configurations—compact, square, and octagonal. Each pavilion had its separate ventilation system; its own restrictions on activities, driven by the type of diseases being treated there; and often its own staff, so as to further limit cross-infection.

A new generation of hospitals was being constructed, and from the

1880s to roughly the 1930s, they often emulated Johns Hopkins. Whether in the booming industrial city of Cincinnati, Ohio, or the sleepy southern town of Jacksonville, Florida, the pavilion plan proved flexible. One reason was that the form was adaptable to local social conditions and medical needs. In Jacksonville, pavilions were constructed not only for public and private patients, male and female patients, but also for white and "colored" patients.[22] By the beginning of the twentieth century, sanitary reform, nutrition improvements, and to a lesser extent medical innovations brought on by the bacteriological revolution had diminished the deadly role of infectious and contagious diseases. Environmental concerns, though, continued to shape the design of America's hospitals well into the twentieth century. Long after bacteriology displaced the miasmic theory of disease transmission, Nightingale's requirements would influence the construction of new hospitals.

American hospital designers continued to be concerned with improving ward ventilation systems and using new technology to ensure patient isolation. They also brought forward other design elements of the early pavilion hospitals. Most importantly, Nightingale honored sun as well as air; so, large windows, open-air porches and verandahs, and sunrooms were popular until the 1920s in general hospitals. These and other sitting spaces, allowed hospital staff to park patients outside to get the fresh air that was believed to help their recovery. When West Penn Hospital moved in 1909 from its 1883 facility, which had full-length porches, architect John L. Beatty was careful to include open porches, a roof garden, and solariums in the new building.[23] Even though Beatty's wheel design looked little like its rustic Victorian predecessor, it reflected the same concerns about environmental conditions that dictated Nightingale's prescriptions.

Johns Hopkins Hospital and the generation of hospitals that emulated it represented a transition between the hospital's past as a public charity and its future as a scientific necessity. Even though the pavilion-plan design relied on a theory of disease transmission that was already under attack in European laboratories, it represented a medicalization of the hospital. As Dell Upton has noted, "the Nightingale system" as constructed at Johns Hopkins and elsewhere "applied a veneer of science to the passive ventilating techniques long used in vernacular buildings." He points out that at Johns Hopkins, an isolating ward "employed interior partitions and individual ventilating systems that crystallized the atmospheric cocoon of the common wards," tying this design to that of contemporary prison buildings as well as of hotels and offices.[24] These changes heralded a new era in medicine. The early hospital was intended for moral edification. The pavilion hospital was designed with social concerns in mind, but with scientific ones increasingly paramount.

A Scientific Approach

The historical irony is that the foundations of modern medicine were formulated in buildings designed according to a competing theory of disease transmission. Inside the pavilions, a generation of European-trained physicians was instituting a new style of medicine. Johns Hopkins inaugurated a scientific style when it initiated a model for American medical education adapted from European practices.[25] Formerly, American doctors had been trained in an apprentice system, now their education was standardized and rationalized, using the hospital clinic as the central mechanism for study. Clinical training emphasized the constant interaction of the undergraduate and graduate medical student with patients undergoing care. On the wards, medical students witnessed the spread of disease, learned the care of specific diseases, and assimilated medical culture. Not only did such changes promote the construction of hospitals, they also dramatically extended the physicians' control over the hospital. Patients still had to be convinced to use the hospital, but in their medical workshop, the physicians reigned supreme, raising their professional status even as they recreated the hospital into a prominent American institution.

Intimately connected with the development of the emerging system for educating doctors was the professionalization of nursing. While the old system depended on ambulatory patients to watch other patients, the professional nurse, so commonly associated with Florence Nightingale and Clara Barton, was trained to supervise more patients and to provide them with a better quality of care. Conversant with the growing arsenal of diagnostic and treatment protocols, she was becoming essential in the development of the medical workshop. Some physicians worried about the nurse becoming a competitor, but gradually these doubts were overcome.[26] It would take until well into the twentieth century before the professional status of nurses would be recognized by state laws as well as by the whole medical community, yet nursing reform established another key link in the modernization of the medical system.

The array of new technologies demanded a sophisticated understanding and education that many physicians did not have the time or the inclination to acquire, and this fostered specialization among practitioners. Gradually, the physicians who had trained on certain machines or in specific procedures were the ones expected to perform those tasks. The general practitioner was redefined as a gatekeeper by whom patients were referred to the physicians with the specialized skills to handle their medical problem. While medicine had always had divisions (mainly based on economics), specialization (and later subspecialization) segmented practitioners while serving as the foundation for increasing public confidence in American medicine. The hospital played a central role in medical education and in the development of the specializations, and by early in the twentieth century the clinical education pioneered at Johns Hopkins had become standard practice. These changes were codified in the Flexner Report of 1910. Abraham Flexner's investigation of medical education validated the hospital-based system and resulted in stringent new standards for medical schools. The foundation of a new era in American medicine had been laid.[27]

Central to the changes in medicine was a revolution in surgery. Operating rooms had rarely been constructed as distinctive spaces in older hospitals, but the practice became mandatory in new hospitals, and they started to be added to older ones in the 1890s. The operating suites represented the culmination of the redesign of the hospital from an imitation of domestic and monastic spaces to a medical workshop. Surgery had come a long way since the beginning of the century, as one example illustrates. In December 1809, Dr. Ephraim McDowell was asked to consult on a difficult pregnancy case. Mrs. Jane Todd Crawford, McDowell quickly realized, was not pregnant but suffering from a large ovarian tumor. McDowell had "never seen so large a substance extracted, nor heard of an attempt or success attending any operation such as this required." Nonetheless, he convinced Mrs. Crawford to travel by horseback sixty miles to his home in Danville, Kentucky, so he could attempt the operation. Anesthesia was not yet available, nor had the concept of antiseptic conditions yet been demonstrated. The surgery was performed in McDowell's home, and the patient endured incredible pain.

Assisted by his nephew, McDowell extracted the very large tumor from his patient, as she sang songs to distract herself from the pain. Further evidence of the fear engendered by surgery was the large group of men waiting outside the door, rope in hand, to hang him if he failed. Given the high mortality rate that attended surgery in the United States at the time, McDowell proved both skillful and lucky. Not only did Mrs. Crawford survive the surgery, but within days McDowell caught her making her own bed![28]

Surgery was dangerous in those days particularly because of the ever-present danger of postsurgical infections, such as gangrene, which would usually kill the patient. Considering the problems presented by the operation, Crawford was fortunate not to become infected from microbes in the room's furnishing, the surgeon's clothes, and the uncovered hands and faces of those in the room; but she was probably better off in McDowell's living room than in a hospital. Isolated in his home, at least she was not moved after the surgery into a ward filled with other postoperative patients. In those wards, the development of gangrene in one patient could signal death for many others.

Surgery results were improved by a series of technological advances. The demonstration of anesthesia in the 1840s and the development of antiseptic, then aseptic, procedures in the 1880s, greatly improved patients' chances of survival from surgery, childbirth, and other procedures that exposed the body to infection. Roentgen's discovery of the x-ray was immediately adapted to medical use. By World War I, virtually all hospitals had installed x-ray machines. These advances further heightened the surgeon's understanding of problems that might be addressed surgically, and this led to a rapid expansion of surgical procedures. In 1899, a report by William Mayo of the Mayo Clinic on 105 gallbladder operations had been rejected by a prominent medical journal because the number of procedures was thought implausible; just five years later, Mayo published an article reporting on one thousand such operations.[29]

The early, elaborately designed operating suites were as much theaters as medical spaces. Operations often were being done for the first time in a region, so many students and other surgeons wanted to watch. In 1886, Dr. D. Hayes Agnew performed a leg operation in the University of Pennsylvania's School of Medicine's operating theater. In the evocative painting by Thomas Eakins that captures that event, over one hundred students crane their necks to get the best perspective as they sit on ascending semicircular rows of wooden benches. Agnew, dressed in his street clothes, works on a patient, while his assistant administers anesthesia. The students are separated from the operation by a short wooden railing that defines the surgical theater. Natural light pours in from the skylights and surrounding windows.

The whole scene suggests a college lecture hall where a professor gives special presentations. And so it was. The new medicine required that medical students experience, first vicariously, then directly, the actual practice of medicine. The operating suite's seats would be filled regularly by students cramming to understand the technical wonders of the emerging science of surgery before they would be asked themselves to perform the procedures. Innovations in science and medicine had provided medicine with tools that allowed for much greater specificity in diagnosis and greater chance of successful intervention. The surgical suite was the most important of these tools.

Specialty Hospitals

Just as the spaces within the hospital became increasingly segmented as specialists reshaped the hospital to meet evolving professional needs, the field of hospitals itself was becoming differentiated. During the last years of the nineteenth century, hospitals were opened that were intended specifically for children, women, pregnant women, orthopaedic patients, patients with contagious diseases, and other special populations that the medical establishment thought needed special care or different spaces for their care.

Children's hospitals are representative of this trend. The concept of a specialty hospital for children first emerged in Europe in the late eighteenth century. After unsuccessfully experimenting with outpatient dispensaries that focused on children's care, some physicians advocated for a specialty hospital. The French were apparently the first to establish such a hospital—Hôpital des Enfants Malades, created in Paris in 1802. The English followed a half-century later in 1852 when the Hospital for Sick Children in Great Ormond Street was established in London. The Americans were close behind the English, with the 1855 founding of Children's Hospital in Philadelphia.[30]

The concept spread very slowly. Boston's Children's Hospital was this nation's second, founded 14 years after Philadelphia's. That same year, 1869, the Foundling Hospital was established in New York. During the 1870s, seven more hospitals were established, including ones in Washington, D.C., St. Louis, Louisville, and Albany. The movement continued, spreading into the nation's heartland during the 1880s. New hospitals were opened in Chicago, Minneapolis, Detroit, and Cincinnati. Almost all of the early hospitals were nonprofit organizations focused on providing care for indigent children. Gradually, as the hospital concept became more acceptable, paying patients were admitted as well.

As medicine more discretely categorized medical expertise, creating specializations based both on disease (cancer and heart specialists) and population (pediatricians and obstetricians), the number of children's hospitals expanded more quickly. In the first twenty years of the twentieth century, new children's hospitals were founded in the west, in Los Angeles, Oakland, and Seattle. Additional hospitals opened in Massachusetts, Pennsylvania, and New York, and children's hospitals spread into southern cities—in Texas, Virginia, North Carolina, Georgia, Tennessee, and Louisiana. By the 1920s, independent children's hospitals and children's units within large general hospitals had opened in most large American cities.

Children's hospitals were rarely initially housed in buildings constructed for that purpose. Instead, as with most general hospitals opened between 1880 and 1930, their founders converted residences, to save money and to prove the experiment of a specialty hospital for children prior to spending real money on a substantial building. When the superintendent of Washington's hospital for children, Mary Rogers, wrote the first overview of children's hospitals in 1894, she noted that Philadelphia's hospital had 12 beds designated for children, and Boston and Detroit had the same, while Washington had 6, San Francisco 4, and Albany 2. She praised a New York hospital, opened in 1887, for having the courage to begin with as many as 50 beds set aside for children.[31]

The number of beds expanded as the size of hospitals grew, but the prime reason for the increase was that hospitals were gradually viewed as being able to respond to the specific needs of children. One important consequence of the germ theory was the development of treatments for some of the deadliest diseases that struck children, such as tuberculosis, scarlet fever, and diphtheria. The improved circumstances of surgery meant that orthopedic conditions, which afflicted many children, were much more likely to be operable than they previously had been. A combination of a half-century of sanitation reform, housing and recreation improvements, and the new technology of medicine led to a dramatic reduction in childhood deaths. While children had accounted for roughly 40 percent of deaths in the 1890s, the proportion had declined to roughly 25 percent by the mid-1920s.

As medicine recognized that specific actions could be taken for children as a special population, the medical specialty of pediatrics emerged. In 1881, Dr. Abraham Jacobi organized the Pediatric Section of the American Medical Society. This organization, along with a host of state and national organizations that followed, represented the staking out of professional turf, the coming together of physicians with similar interests, and a powerful professionalizing influence on the medical care of children. The number of pediatricians remained very small; only about 100 physicians identified themselves as such in the 1910s. But their influence was significant given, their involvement in "creating the institutions that marked the development of this specialty in America: children's hospitals, children's clinics, professional pediatric associations, professorships separate from obstetrics and gynecology, and new journals devoted to children's diseases."[32] Pediatrics represented another way that children were understood to have different medical needs and problems. The specialty hospitals built to serve them reflected those differences.

Designs for children's hospitals combined the continuing fears of old problems with hospitals and glimpses of the modern medical machine. Designers were searching for the right combination of style and function for the patients boarded at a children's hospital. They accepted that children represented a special case, different from adults. As noted architect Edward F. Stevens wrote, "In planning for a children's hospital . . . we have new conditions that do not exist in any of the other departments."[33] Architects not only supported their separation from adults but also adapted the hospital's design to the experts' perceptions of the children's needs.

Although much about the arrangement of children's hospitals was similar to what was being done in general hospitals, a few aspects were very different. First, the designs were carefully adapted to safeguard the children and to establish medical routine. A rigorous admissions process supplemented by easily accessible isolation rooms guarded against contagion, one of the greatest fears of the time. In an age of tuberculosis and multiple other infectious diseases, such concerns were only prudent, yet the emphasis on contagion also allowed medical staff to limit family visits and maintain strict control over the interaction of patients and parents. Second, children's hospitals were often built with large roofed porches where children could be exposed to fresh air and parents could come to view their children from afar. Porches had been typical on late-nineteenth-century general hospitals as well, but they were retained as part of children's hospitals much longer.

Third, while general hospitals were moving away from the domestic model, designers of the largest and smallest of children's hospitals attempted to maintain the fiction of the home within the institutional setting. When Mary Rogers presented her overview of children's hospitals to a public health conference in 1894, she reminded her audience that the institutions had been embraced by parents because they did not seem the same to them as general hospitals. She related that mothers had repeatedly told her that they would never take their child to a "big" hospital for fear of leaving the child in the care of strangers.[34] Playrooms, parlors, libraries, and other domestic rooms were often included in early-twentieth-century children's hospitals, as is evidenced by examples in contemporary architectural books. For children, a homelike atmosphere was deemed appropriate in the minds of designers, trustees, and medical staff, long after the scientific hospital had turned to the factory or laboratory for models.

Children's hospitals were only one example of the development of specialty hospitals, but they are representative of the ways in which the needs of a specific population were translated into new medical practices and specially tailored medical facilities. On features like the rehabilitation rooms in orthopedic hospitals and the private rooms in the mental health facilities, architects worked with medical staffs to develop distinct characteristics for these hospitals. However, they ultimately represented another wave in the general acceptance of the hospital, as Americans embraced the new medicine.

Learning to Love the Hospital

Although the number of hospitals was rapidly expanding, most continued to face the financial challenges that have always plagued American nonprofit organizations. From the organization of Pennsylvania Hospital onward, hospitals have struggled to provide services to those least able to pay for those services. They have depended upon charitable contributions, voluntary service by physicians, and the supplement of a few paying patients to keep their precarious finances solvent. Pennsylvania Hospital, for instance, took a half-century to complete their buildings, constantly shoring up their finances in the face of too many poor people in need of treatment and not enough contributions.

Americans came to accept, even revere the hospital by the mid-twentieth century. Hospital fund campaigns were standard practice in cities and towns around the nation. The local hospital became a focus of philanthropy, voluntarism, and activism by fraternal clubs and society clubs. The financial difficulties never subsided, but the number of hospitals continued to expand and the resources available to hospital administrators also grew.

By 1960, Americans had embraced the hospital as the site of care for their serious medical problems. Even as the average length of stay in a hospital declined from 48 days in 1904 to just under 8 days in 1960, the number of admissions skyrocketed from roughly 1 million to almost 23 million. Virtually all of the births and approximately half the deaths occurred in the nation's 5,500+ hospitals. In the 1930s, the creation of Blue Cross and Blue Shield provided a growing number of Americans with private health insurance. In 1940, only 9 percent of Americans had some form of health insurance, while that figure had reached almost 70 percent by 1960.[35] Middle-class, then working-class Americans who could not formerly afford hospital services increasingly received private insurance through their employers or came under expanding governmental programs.

People did not go to the hospital just because doing so had become affordable. Hospitals had become accepted necessities for everyone. So much so that the federal government felt compelled to support their construction. In the 1940s, the federal government began assisting hospitals; the Hill-Burton Act of 1947 provided funds for hospital construction. This legislation would support the construction or expansion of hundreds of hospitals nationwide but particularly in smaller towns or underserved cities. Federal funds reinforced the hospital's centrality in the healthcare system. Two decades later, the enactment of Medicare and Medicaid in the 1960s dramatically increased the number of patients who received government subsidies and the government's role in overseeing the healthcare system.[36] Gradually, the public used the hospital for a wider and wider range of services, coming to view it as an essential local institution.

MEDICINE MOVES TO THE MALL

The reasons for this change in public perceptions are complicated and not fully understood. Charles Rosenberg, in his magisterial study of the hospital's rise, notes that the conventional view is that Americans embraced the hospital out of "no more than a natural response to the new technical resources of the medical profession allied with the changed domestic ecology of an increasingly urban population." However, as he goes on to say, this view has "a number of difficulties." Such a story of inevitable change ignores the hospital's promotional efforts and the tale of continuing patient resistance to the change. Also, while middle-class Americans "certainly did entertain a growing faith in the efficacy of medicine," the change has largely been unexamined by scholars. Even if they would examine this changing faith: "Attitudes are difficult to evaluate in the present; past attitudes are even more elusive."[37] Patient resistance to the change was partially driven by concerns over the loss of control and comfort, suggesting that the path from marginal charitable care to medical necessity was far from straight.

The shift of the patient from home to hospital certainly reinforced a loss of control, even a loss of identity. As a pioneer in the need for home treatment of the mentally ill noted, "At home, even though he was a sick man, the patient retained his identity and the sense of belonging; he was with his family and he felt secure because he was still in the community he knew and which he understood. In hospital, the patient is an enforced member of a group living in an entirely artificial environment bearing no relation to anything approaching ordinary home life, but where everything is strange and often frightening."[38] The buildings themselves reinforced the loss of control, the sense of strangeness, and the fear of the unknown. These shifts suggest that present-day attempts to redesign the hospital in a more patient-centered manner have deep roots.

As Rosenberg noted, patients resisted the requirements that they leave the house and heed the advice of their physicians to enter the hospital. A prime reason may have been that the shift in place represented far more than a new location. All patients, poor, wealthy and middle class, gave up control over their illnesses to the physicians, who competed for the privilege to care for them, and the nurses who oversaw their daily routine. Journalist Winfred Rhoades related a story of a well-off woman admitted to a hospital for the treatment of a back disorder. The woman had gone into the hospital "in the spirit not only of trust, but of eager cooperation." However, her physicians had little desire for cooperation. They placed her in a bed "in what was considered the proper position to bring about the needed adjustment," and left her there without comment. On the third day, her specialist finally appeared, long after the patient had lost the "blind faith" she had previously held toward his competence or caring. She cried out, "The one who does the suffering has a right to understand." Rhoades criticized the physician for "nonchalant professionalism" bordering on "utter indifference to her mental state." The new hospital routine emphasized the ill person's passivity.[39]

While all patients relinquished control when entering the hospital, they were not all treated in the same section of the hospital. The broad divide between rich and poor was represented in the differences between paying and charity patients. The voluntary general hospital had long served paying as well as dependent patients. Antebellum hospitals depended on the paying patients for financial support. Some paying patients, such as sailors, who were covered by one of the nation's first health insurance programs, were treated little different from the charity patients. Others, such as wealthy bachelors or merchant travelers, were allowed to bring servants with them, to supplement hospital food with their own wines and extras, and avoided the compensatory duties other patients had to perform, such as cleaning the hospital and caring for fellow patients. They also received better care, being treated by the more prominent physicians. These patients remained a minority, outside the social mission of the hospital, until the scientific revolution in medicine began to reshape the hospital.

As hospital environments improved, physicians began encouraging wealthy mothers-to-be to have their births in hospitals, further increasing specialized units. Also, surgeries that would have been completed either at home or in a physician's office were now moved to the hospital. The wealthy expected a different level of care than hospitals had traditionally provided the poor, recreating the two-tiered system of care. Private patients were housed in single rooms with domestic settings. Their rooms had bureaus and sitting chairs, amenities intended to make them feel at home.[40] They had easy access (sometimes sole access) to conservatories, sun rooms, verandahs, and roof porches. They often had private nurses and almost always were cared for by their private physician. In such ways they maintained their privacy while benefiting from the increasing sophistication of hospital care.

Charity wards were less sumptuous in decoration and services. In the

1920s, attempts were made to give ward patients greater privacy by changing from a "perimeter" to a "Rigs" configuration. In the former, the beds are each perpendicular to the wall. In the "Rigs ward," named after the Copenhagen hospital where it originated, the beds are grouped in semiprivate bays created by glazed glass dividers. The beds, instead of being against the wall, are set in twos parallel to the wall, each set facing another set.[41] Later, the glass dividers were turned into walls and a new room type, the semiprivate room (or ward), was create. The social tensions produced by the physical segregation of wealthy patients in their private rooms and poor in their wards were reflected in several articles that appeared in popular periodicals, asking for a "homelike hospital" or a "hospital like a hotel."[42]

As new avenues of funding opened up, they restructured patient expectations. The large ward was still the image most commonly associated with the hospital at the turn of the century. As we have seen, though, in the 1920s the 20-bed ward shrank to the 4-bed ward, and then to the 2-bed semiprivate room in the 1940s and 1950s.[43] The private, or at least the semiprivate room, was gradually viewed by most as a reasonable standard for all private patients. Public hospitals retained larger wards for economic reasons, as evidenced by the 24-bed wards common at Los Angeles County Hospital in the 1960s. The postwar building boom propelled by Hill-Burton funds simply reinforced the shrinking of wards and proliferation of semiprivate rooms. By 1971, architect Michael Bobrow could write an overview of current nursing units that argued that "the concept of the all single-bed room hospital is now becoming widely accepted."[44] Few mid-century hospitals, however, went to strictly private rooms, because they were too expensive, too staff intensive, and administrators found that some patients disliked being alone in the hospital.

The Vertical Hospital

The hospital was undergoing another transformation, from a horizontal pavilion plan to a compact vertical design. The discovery and validation of the germ theory of disease transmission provided additional impetus for rethinking the basic arrangement of the hospital. A 1939 article in *Architectural Record* declared, "Hospital designers have discarded . . . the 'pavilion' or 'continental' type—which results in one- or two-story buildings with their various departments strung along corridors. The trend of hospital design is toward a compact, multistory plan, which is at once less expensive and more elastic to operate."[45] The pavilion had lasted long after bacteriology had proven its basis incorrect. However, new urban hospitals rarely had the luxurious expanse of land necessary for one- or two-story pavilions. Caspar Morris, a physician, had argued as early as the design competition for Johns Hopkins Hospital that a city hospital "must be adapted to the requirements of city life."[46] Finally, fifty years after Hopkins opened, hospitals across the nation started becoming more compactly constructed.

The early modern hospitals were designed as stacks of pavilions with sophisticated ventilation systems that maintained isolation. By the 1920s, when they became standard practice in most cities, this design was viewed as more efficient and more suitable for scientific medicine. Architect Isadore Rosenfield described the typical arrangement of the hospital in his 1947 book on hospital design: "The average hospital in any large city is a vertical hospital. It generally begins at the bottom with the administrative offices. On the next floor it might have physiotherapy and the other diagnostic and therapeutic facilities. On these would be imposed the wards, on top of which would come the semi-private rooms and then the private rooms; on the very top, normally, would be the operating department."[47] Elevators, improved artificial lighting, steel and concrete structures, and other engineering advancements allowed for taller, larger hospitals that bundled all the medical activities into a single shell. The simple patterns of early American hospitals, with their long corridors and large wards, had given way to spatial differentiation and institutional complexity where the hospital was segmented into an ever-expanding number of sections, each providing a separate but interrelated service.

Architects had been involved in designing hospitals from the very earliest hospitals. However, with the advent first of the pavilion, then particularly the vertical hospital, the complexities of the design challenges resulted in healthcare becoming an architectural specialization. Increasingly, a small group of experts provided advice to their more generalist architectural colleagues about the intricacies of hospital construction. The European hospital design literature had exploded with the advent of the pavilion concept in the late eighteenth century, but American architects only slowly joined the discussion. After a few scattered writings on hospital construction and design prior to the Civil War, the campaign for pavilion hospitals resulted in a growing number of articles and books after 1870. These proved the beginning of a large volume of works that increased throughout the twentieth century, producing numerous guides, compilations, building typologies, and case studies. Architects active in the hospital field here and in Europe wrote most of the articles and books. Such classics as Edward F. Stevens's *The American Hospital in the Twentieth Century* (1928), Isadore Rosenfield's *Hospitals: An Integrated Design* (1947), and Louis Redstone's *Hospitals and Healthcare Facilities* (1960), joined periodic volumes published by *Architectural Record, Architecture,* and the American Hospital Association. They chronicled the growing complexity of the buildings, the move towards functionalism, and eventually, the criticisms that led to reform after the 1960s.[48]

In addition, architects such as Edward Stevens were called upon to design hospitals throughout North America. As architectural historian Annmarie Adams has reported, the firm of Stevens and Lee emerged as the leading designer of hospitals in the early twentieth century. These architects joined with a small group of physicians, including S. S. Goldwater, superintendent of Mount Sinai Hospital in New York City, who served as medical consultants on hospital projects, influencing generations of designers and hospital managers.[49] They largely convinced their colleagues to repudiate the pavilion and to embrace the vertical hospital. They participated in long, intense discussions of the right size and shape for a nursing unit, the appropriateness of color in the hospital, the role of outpatient clinics, and the many other debates that ensued as the modern hospital became the complex institution of the present day.

Between the 1890s and the 1940s, American hospitals' exterior façades evolved from highlighting the hospital's civic institutionalism to reflecting the hospitals' scientific functionalism. Hospital exteriors were slow to manifest the scientific revolution occurring inside, perhaps because of the public's lingering fears of the hospital as an institution. Annmarie Adams has demonstrated that this was an international phenomenon. Hospitals constructed after the era of the pavilion style and before World War II were "modern in spatial attitudes," but not necessarily in the way they looked. The architects clothed "modern plans in historic dress in order to smooth the effects of social change." Only gradually could society accept the hospital as a "modern factory of healing." Good medical care was still associated with the home, not the hospital; and even with the advent of new scientific marvels, those attitudes only slowly evolved.[50]

Hospitals around the nation went through similar transitions. California Hospital in Los Angeles offers a good example. First in 1926 and again in 1955 and 1971, new additions expanded the hospital. Successively, modernist architects stripped away more of the civic presence and decorative symbols, replacing them with a functional façade. The hospital was no longer a symbol of paternal beneficence. Instead, the buildings represented medicine's scientific application and efficient success. Edward F. Stevens compared designing the hospital to the efficiencies then being sought in American businesses:

> Hospital planning demands the same careful thought that is the foundation of any modern successful business enterprise. It is essential in the shoe factory, the paper mill, or the business establishment to so plan that the raw materials may be assembled and the finished product delivered with the fewest possible intervening motions. In the hospital, the patient, the food and the treatment may be termed the raw material. Whatever conduces to recovery, the convalescent being the finished product, is of business importance in the hospital. The care, the comfort, the convenience and the food, together with the treatment, are the processes of manufacture.[51]

Time management studies of hospital personnel had begun influencing hospital designs soon after Frederick Taylor popularized them in business. The more complex the building, the more mechanical the care, the easier the analogies between industry and medicine became. Striving to maintain comfort and care in the routine of the medical workshop was increasingly difficult.

The buildings themselves reflected the emphasis on efficiency and effectiveness. In 1949, the American Institute of Architects held a seminar on hospitals during their annual convention. Jacque Norman noted at that conference that, while he was trained in the tradition of Greek and Roman classicism, "I must concede too, and hardily endorse functional design for hospitals. . . . [F]unctional design best correlates these varied activities such as nursing education, intern and resident physician education, research and various adjunct or service facilities of the hospital into a unit offering ultimately, proper care for the patient."[52] Only a functional design could encompass the diverse and complex roles that the hospital had assumed incrementally over the previous half-century. Ornamentation was omitted, leaving scientific rationality as the structure's visible symbol. Hospital after hospital was designed in this fashion.

Federal legislation supporting the construction of hospitals signaled another postwar burst in construction. While many of these hospitals were simple modernist boxes of 2–5 stories, a growing number of urban hospitals stretched toward the sky. In a reversal of nineteenth-century doctrine, hospitals were built to last for generations, and one or two stories was no longer viewed as the optimal height. Twelve-, 13-, even 20-story hospitals mushroomed in city after city. New York's Cornell Hospital (1930s) was an early example of the skyscraper hospital, but by the 1960s and 1970s the form was found across the nation in the largest cities. Even in the notoriously horizontal cityscape of Southern California, 20-story Los Angeles County Hospital was joined by skyscraper buildings for Cedars-Sinai, California, UCLA, and other leading hospitals.

Chaotic Growth

Size and efficiency, though, constantly collided with innovation. In hospitals around the nation, carefully established systems of communication and organization were upset by developments in biomedicine and medical technology. The hospital failed to stay within the bounds of any one static design. It had to keep growing, expanding, and changing, even as it searched for stasis.

Additions to Santa Barbara Cottage Hospital during the 1910s exemplify the incremental emergence of the modern hospital.[53] The hospital's original structure was a Victorian-style, two-story, renovated home. In 1913, an additional three-story structure designed by E. Russell Ray expanded the number of beds while improving service facilities, as well as incorporating a modern x-ray room and operating room. In 1918, a wing was added for maternity patients only, so the hospital could compete with midwives and others who until then had birthed most babies at home. McCulloch Hospital in San Diego advertised that it offered its maternity patients "every advantage of modern science" yet in a "modern and home-like" facility, trying to combat the competitive edge that midwives delivering at home had over the sterile hospital. By 1921, Cottage had 16 doctors offering 10 specialty clinics.

Science, defined in terms of both research and practice, drove the development of the hospital. In 1919, the Cottage Hospital's Memorial Metabolic Clinic, designed by Winsor Soule, was opened, focusing on nephritis, gout, and diabetes research and treatment. Hospitals had long served as sites for clinical research, but the modern hospital was inextricably connected to biomedicine. (In 1924 in San Diego, the Scripps Metabolic Clinic, renamed Scripps Clinic and Research Foundation in 1955, was founded with similar research aspirations.) Within hospitals or at independent facilities, research had become part of medicine's mission. Also in 1919, Cottage Hospital added a third wing, for the x-ray department. In 30 years, Santa Barbara Cottage Hospital evolved from a small clinic in a house to a large modern hospital; and the building style shifted to represent this change, from a domestic setting to a mission-style exterior, then to a larger civic-style building.

However, expansion had negative consequences for hospitals. Buildings turned into medical complexes, as the space needs of technology and treatment continually expanded. Often, the apparently chaotic spatial conditions that eventually developed in hospitals were not the fault of any single decision, but happened because, just as with the cities and towns in which the hospitals stood, rarely had there been a grand plan that could cover all the contingencies. Sometimes smaller existing buildings in the surrounding area were converted as clinics and treatment centers or administrative and medical offices. Other times, additional wings were added. Sometimes, the hospital was razed and a new building erected; but in most cases, hospital associations could not afford complete makeovers, so they grew haphazardly. Ironically, even as the additions complicated the space and obscured passageways, the continual expansion of hospitals was viewed by most Americans as a symbol of success, since these institutions represented the burgeoning biomedical knowledge they expected to keep them alive. Only when community members were compelled to find their way through the hospital maze were they confronted with the paradox that the nation's perhaps most technologically sophisticated institution was housed in perhaps its most confusing buildings.

In 1893, Mary Hitchcock Memorial Hospital opened in Hanover, New Hampshire, the sleepy rural location of Dartmouth College and Medical

School. The hospital was a gift from Hiram Hitchcock in memory of his wife, Mary Maynard Hitchcock. The 36-bed hospital consisted of a central administration building and three pavilions. In the words of a contemporary, for roughly $200,000, Hitchcock was able to create a hospital that was "equipped surgically and medically in accordance with the strictest requirements of modern hospital construction," with the comforts of home, since "it is elegantly furnished, surrounded by broad lawns."[54] Not simply a hospital, but "an ideal home" for the acutely and chronically ill. However, the original building was almost immediately too small. Two new wards were added in 1913. A nurses' home, student infirmary, kitchen, dining room, and more personnel quarters followed during the 1920s. In the middle of the Depression, the hospital received more than 2,000 subscriptions to help pay for a new wing that would house laboratories, operating rooms, and facilities for the expanding specialties of pediatrics and obstetrics. The money also would pay for another nurses' residence, a new power plant, and additions to the original patient pavilions. In less than 40 years, the "ideal home" had matured into a modern medical facility with an increasingly complex physical plant. By 1940, the hospital had 164 beds, 128 more than in 1893.

A decade later, the changes were even more dramatic. In 1952, the hospital totally changed its appearance when Faulkner House was added, aided by a million-dollar donation from its namesake's widow, Hill-Burton funds, and community subscriptions. The 1952 addition was a basement with four stories, expanded to eight stories in the 1960s, and a three-story wing. Administrative offices were consolidated, new operating rooms opened, medical office space dramatically expanded, and 120 new patient beds added. It completely change the hospital's appearance because it was situated directly in front of the entrance to the hospital and completely obscured the previous hospital. The horizontal-plan 1893 building was suddenly transformed into a modern-style glass and steel tower. The older, civic look of the hospital was stripped away and replaced with a functional appearance.

Postwar hospitals constantly had to grow to meet increasing patient demand and to accommodate the expanding arsenal of medical technology. Most grew by adding buildings or wings or floors, a solution that disrupted pedestrian pathways. Mary Hitchcock Memorial Hospital became ever more complex. Eventually, as in many other hospitals, patients were instructed to follow colored tapes on the floor to find their way through the

THE MEDICAL WORKSHOP

maze of departments and offices. Few buildings were destroyed in the search for more and more space; new ones were simply added on to the back, the side, the top, even the bottom. Senator Norris Cotton spearheaded successful efforts to get a $3 million federal appropriation to construct a prototype regional cancer center at Mary Hitchcock. The center, later named for the senator, was constructed under the hospital's parking lot, although later funding allowed for a two-story addition above ground.

By 1980, this hospital had become a behemoth stretching out in every direction, surrounded by a dozen smaller buildings, and reconceptualized institutionally into the Dartmouth-Hitchcock Medical Center, a confederation of Dartmouth Medical School, Mary Hitchcock Memorial Hospital, the Hitchcock Clinic, and the Veterans Administration Hospital in nearby White River Junction, Vermont. The original 1893 hospital had been completely gobbled up by the various additions. Space was so crunched inside that closets were regularly used as offices. Patients were constantly confused by the interior maze of offices, basement corridors, and bridges between additions. For instance, women typically gave birth on the third floor of one building and recovered near their babies on the fifth floor of another building. The facilities at Mary Hitchcock and in hospitals around the world confused patients, confounded practitioners, and resulted in a growing rumble of disapproval.

Clouds of Criticism

In these complex medical establishments, healthcare's ability to solve illness and stop the ravages of disease seemed limitless. Physicians became the society's new magicians, armed with magic potions (for instance, antibiotics), arcane spells (medical terminology), and terrifying machines (the deafening booms of the MRI chamber). Americans came to honor and trust medical practitioners in a way they did no other professionals. Expectations rose to unattainable levels. "When a doctor has to tell a patient that there is no specific remedy for his condition, [the patient] is apt to feel affronted, or to wonder if his doctor is keeping abreast of the times."[55] The image of physicians as modern magicians was reinforced by television shows, like *Dr. Kildare*, *Marcus Welby, M.D.*, and *ER*, which have portrayed physicians as the ultimate warriors against death. And the hospital was where their wonders were performed.

However, beginning in the 1960s, a new type of criticism of the hospital began to coalesce. The very qualities of the twentieth century hospital that had made it so appealing, so dominant an aspect of twentieth-century life, have in the last four decades become the focus of intense criticism. Critics complain not only about aspects of medical practice but about the failure of the facilities where they are occurring.

With the triumph of specialization came the criticism that healthcare had been fractured among a plethora of experts who never made contact with the "whole" patient, or each other. Patients were "turfed" from service to service. In this mode, hospital "transport" became a crucial aspect of building design as patients were shuttled from one diagnostic technology to another, rarely seeing "the doctor." Attempts to merely situate diagnostic equipment near patients, so they could be moved as short a space as possible, ran up against the growing space needs of the larger and larger machines. The impersonal and bureaucratic hospital, in its effort to cure, had lost the capacity to care, said critics. Rather than seeing hospitals as institutions in which miracle cures took place, some even went so far as to suggest that contemporary hospitals, like their nineteenth-century predecessors, were dangerous places where the sick would be further sickened. Radical critics such as Ivan Illich suggested that a ubiquitous feature of modern hospitals was iatrogenesis (which *Stedman's Medical Dictionary* politely defines as "Denoting an unfavorable response to therapy, induced by the therapeutic effort itself").[56]

Given such circumstances, many observers asserted that the hospital had failed to achieve the lofty expectations of the first half of the twentieth century. This critique was part of a larger attack on biomedicine and the biomedical model. Medicine had failed to control disease and it was relatively ineffective in addressing the predominance of chronic disease. Further, the hospital was poorly suited to address the medical problems implicit in the epidemiological transition from infectious disease to the chronic systemic diseases of the second half of the twentieth century. Hospital costs skyrocketed while basic health indicators changed little, or, as was the case with infant mortality in some locales, actually worsened. Often towering over inner

THE MEDICAL WORKSHOP

cities, hospitals had become isolated from the communities in which they were situated, symbols of elite science and medicine but out of touch with the social world of disease and illness. The hospital had come to be viewed as a "mixed blessing, a technological and bureaucratic brontosaurus with an enormous appetite, an inadequate heart, and a minute social brain."[57] Americans felt a deep ambivalence about the hospital, and more particularly about the reductionist, technology-centered medicine that it had come to embody. Scientific medicine was both eagerly sought by an expectant public and, at the same time, perceived to be deeply alienating.

Mall Medicine

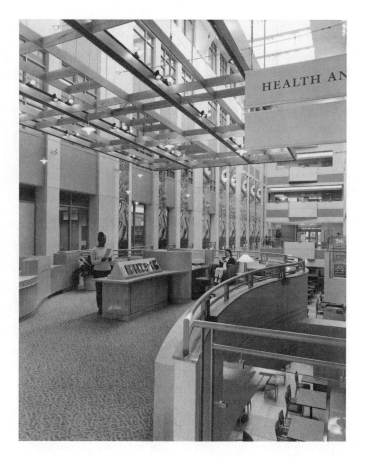

Kalamazoo, Michigan, 2001. In Bronson Methodist Hospital, architects Shepley Bulfinch Richardson and Abbott created "corridors of light," skylit atriums that serve as a consumer service mall running from the parking lot, through the medical office building, into the ambulatory care center. Along the way one can do some banking, grab a sandwich, or enjoy the indoor garden. *Photograph by Peter Mauss, courtesy of Shepley Bulfinch Richardson and Abbott and Esto Photographics.*

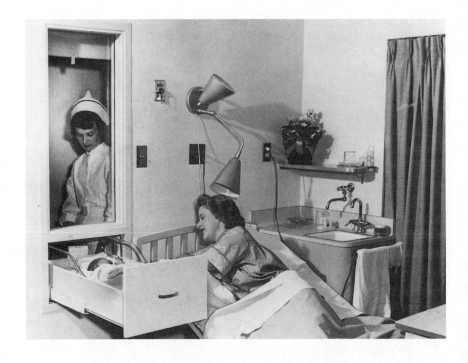

Los Angeles, 1953. The mechanization of the mid-twentieth-century hospital is exemplified in this maternity room at Kaiser Foundation Medical Center. A sliding drawer moves the baby from a bassinet behind the glass to the mother's waiting arms. The mother's access to the baby is improved, compared to communal nurseries located less conveniently, while the baby is shielded from the "unhealthy" attention of visitors. *Courtesy of the University of Southern California, on behalf of the USC Library Department of Special Collections.*

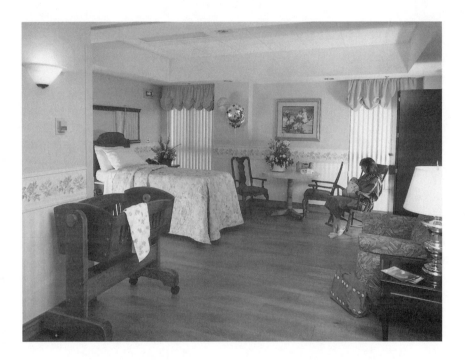

Miami, Florida, 1986. In response to patients' complaints about the sterility of the hospital environment, hospitals created homey birth and delivery suites. This spacious room at South Miami Hospital, designed by The Ritchie Organization, keeps state-of-the-art technology close at hand while accommodating family and friends in an atmosphere more like home than hospital. *Courtesy of the Baptist Health Systems of South Florida.*

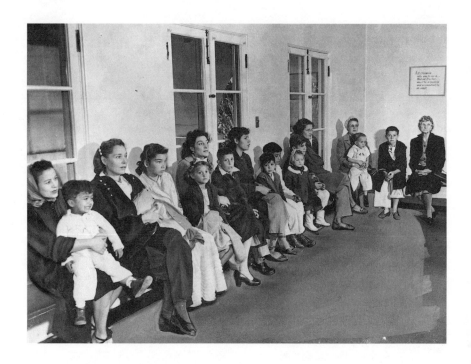

Los Angeles, 1945. Until the 1960s, most hospital outpatient clinics were the stepchildren of inpatient medicine. They were used almost exclusively by poor people and so were often placed in the basement or least desirable location in the hospital or off site altogether. A few clinics found benefactors, as this one did in the actress Marion Davies. *Courtesy of the University of Southern California, on behalf of the USC Library Department of Special Collections.*

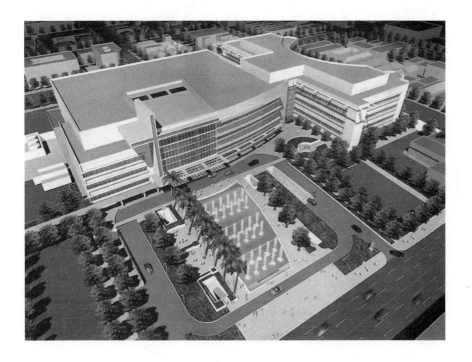

Santa Monica, California, 2001. In St. John's Associate Architects' patient-centered redesign of St. John's Health Center, modeled here, the main entrance leads directly into a diagnostic and treatment facility that includes ambulatory care, surgery rooms, and diagnostic services. *Courtesy of St. John's Health Center.*

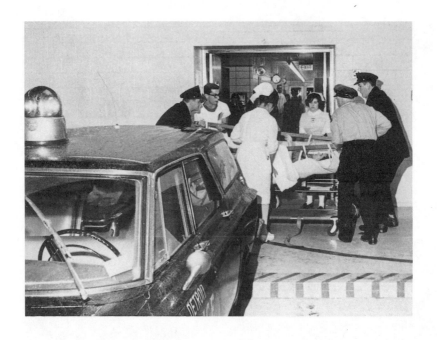

Detroit, 1950s. Mid-twentieth-century emergency rooms were designed for extreme cases arriving by ambulance, not the variety of cases, including many walk-ins, that they now see. The atmosphere was typically entirely functional, lacking the consumer-friendly amenities more common today. *Courtesy of the National Libarary of Medicine, Bethesda, Maryland.*

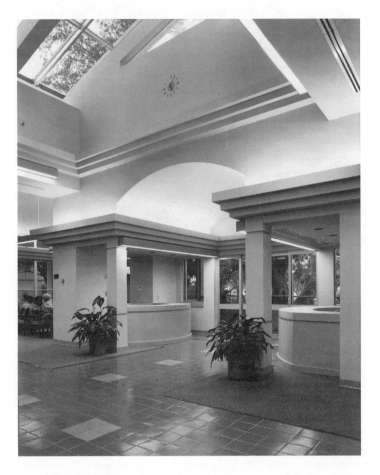

Miami, Florida, 1986. At Miami Baptist Memorial, the "Emergency Center," designed by The Ritchie Organization, has more of a hotel-like ambience, intended
to be welcoming and comfortable for patients and family members. *Photograph by
Robert Mikrut, courtesy of TRO/The Ritchie Organization and Baptist Health Systems of South Florida.*

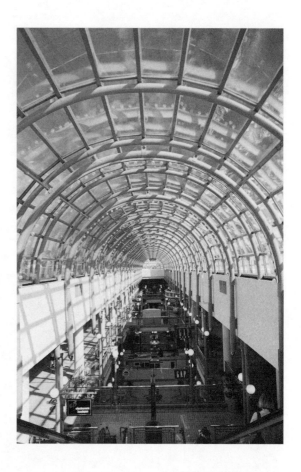

Los Angeles, 2000; Lebanon, New Hampshire, 1992. That the design principles of shopping malls are being used in new hospital construction is obvious in a comparison of Los Angeles's Westside Pavilion Shopping Center (*above*), designed by Jon Jerde Associates, opened in 1985, and the Dartmouth-Hitchcock Medical Center (*right*), designed by Shepley Bulfinch Richardson and Abbott in 1992. *Photographs by Beverlie Conant Sloane (2000), and Jean Smith courtesy of Shepley Bulfinch Richardson and Abbott.*

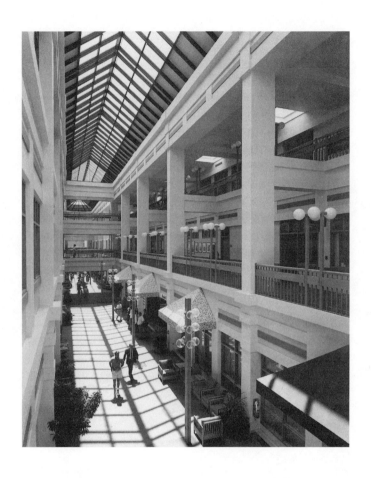

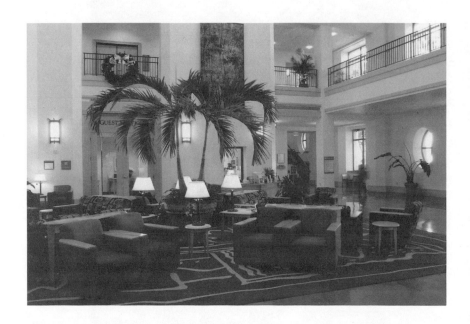

Orlando, 1997; La Jolla, 1993. From Florida Hospital's Celebration Health (*above*), designed by architect Robert A. M. Stern with patient architectural layout by NBBJ, to California's Thornton Hospital (*right*), by Stone, Marraccini, and Patterson, the hotel has served as a model for hospital designers. Both Thornton's soaring, glass-enclosed atrium and Celebration Health's comfortably appointed entrance lobby are devoid of signs of medicine. *Photographs by Matt Jacques, courtesy of Florida Hospital Celebration Health; and David Hewitt and Anne Garrison, courtesy of UCSD Healthcare.*

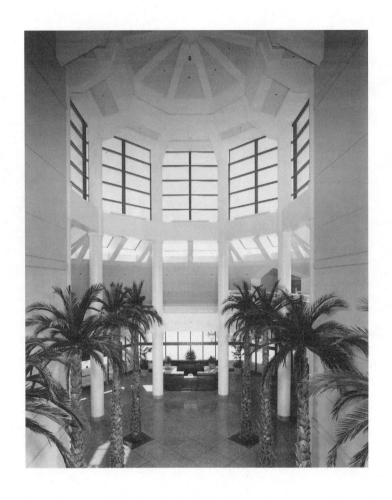

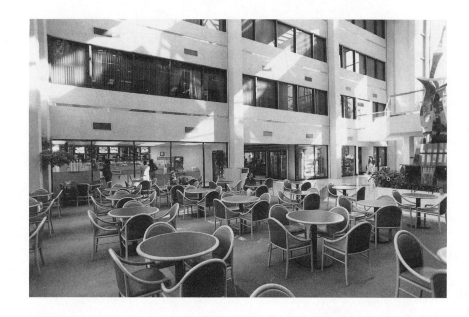

Dallas, Texas, 1974. The atrium in Medical City Dallas Hospital provides a respite from the heaviness of the concrete structure. The tables and surrounding retail stores are lit from skylights and a wall of glass. The hospital is surrounded by medical offices and other services, constituting the nation's first self-proclaimed medical mall, Medical City. *Photograph by Ira Montgomery, courtesy of Medical City Dallas Hospital.*

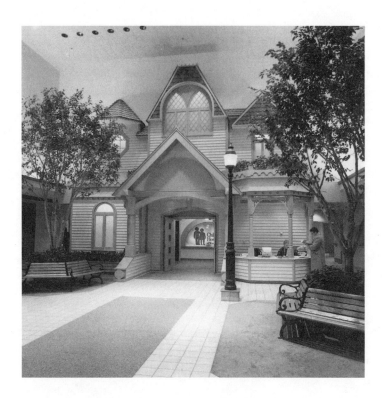

Milwaukee, Wisconsin, 1988. Henningson, Durham and Richardson, architects, are reconfiguring Children's Hospital of Wisconsin, an older, stack hospital, into a more accessible, inviting structure. A Victorian house façade, modeled on the hospital's first home, was constructed in the hospital's lobby to welcome patients and their families. *Courtesy of Children's Hospital of Wisconsin.*

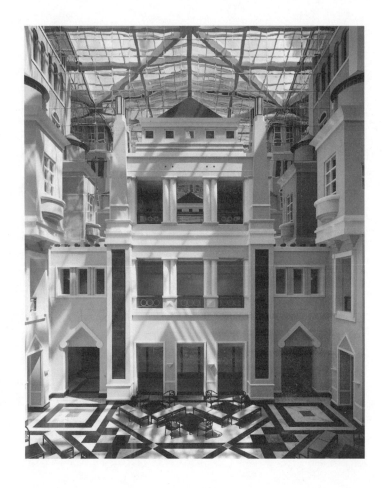

Fort Worth, Texas, 1990. Improved circulation is combined with entertainment in architect David Schwarz's fantasy design for the atrium of Cook–Fort Worth Children's Hospital, an example of a medical space designed for the special type of patient it treats. *Photograph by Michael O. Houlihan, Hedrich-Blessing Photographers, courtesy of David M. Schwarz, Architectural Services.*

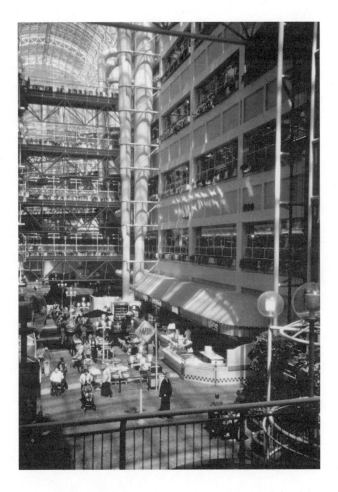

Edmonton, Canada, 1983–86. No architect of hospitals has been more experimental than Zeidler Roberts Partners, whose designs exhibit the lighting and interior atmosphere of a shopping mall by having plenty of public spaces and well-marked circulation systems to ease patients' navigation of the hospital. An example is the Walter C. McKenzie Health Sciences Center. *Photograph by Annmarie Adams, courtesy of Annmarie Adams.*

TWO /   Humanizing the Hospital

E ven burdened with an increasingly complex physical plan, Hanover, New Hampshire's Mary Hitchcock Memorial Hospital represented the continuing efforts by American healthcare providers to balance scientific innovation with patient care. The place was well known locally for having physicians who took the extra moment, nurses who knew just what was bothering a patient, and a large volunteer staff from the community. However, their efforts were increasingly undermined by the physical spaces within which they worked. The hospital's maze of buildings confused, irritated, and alienated just about everyone. Patients waited in a corridor on a stretcher to have an x-ray. Visitors got lost on the way to visit a friend. Physicians had a closet for an office. Nurses used makeshift spaces for examination rooms. Everyone was forced to cope with dark spaces and crowded places. The experience was eroding the hospital staff's relationship with its patients. Even the warmness of the staff could not overcome the coldness of the hospital itself; the physical spaces were neither patient-centered nor visitor friendly. That changed in 1991.

Ninety-eight years after Mary Hitchcock Hospital opened, former Surgeon General C. Everett Koop and other celebrants inaugurated Dartmouth-Hitchcock Medical Center.[1] Mary Hitchcock Hospital stood empty, after months of anticipation and weeks of moving machines, supplies, and finally patients into the new facility. The new hospital was full—of patients and expectations. Few visitors were prepared for the spaciousness, light, and amenities of the new building. Patients and visitors who had previously had to follow colored tape on the corridor floors of Mary Hitchcock to find their way around were startled to see cheerful awnings inscribed with "Admissions," "X-ray," and other department names along the new hospital's mall. As one walked along the mall, looking at art on the walls, glimpsing trees and clouds through walls of windows and a ceiling of skylights, the eye was drawn outside the hospital, then into the medical workplaces, without any loss of a sense of familiarity and comfort. The light, bright atmosphere was inviting instead of intimidating, and was certainly dramatically different from the low ceilings and dark corridors of the old hospital.

Dartmouth-Hitchcock's most dramatic feature is its mall. Explicitly drawing from shopping mall spaces, architects Lloyd Acton and Neil Smith, of the firm of Shepley Bulfinch Richardson and Abbott, designed a circulation system that doubles as a communal space, filled with places to sit and watch as well as 10,000 square feet of retail activity. The new medical center is intended to include inpatient and outpatient services, a medical school, and research facilities. In the future, elements of the Dartmouth Medical School and additional research facilities will be added to the center. The complex uses the mall as a spine from which expansion will occur, hopefully overcoming the maze-like effect from which so many older hospitals suffer.

The mall also offers amenities to patients, staff, and visitors. Benches and chairs allow visitors to wait and patients to rest in a space three stories tall and flooded with light from the glass and girder roof. The retail space, located off the mall on a short side corridor, was born of necessity, since the new hospital is seven miles from downtown Hanover. Patients, visitors, and staff needed services, so the architects planned for them within the new hospital. They could not have imagined how many extra benefits would accrue from that decision. The staff loves the food court. At Sbarro they can pick up a pizza, while their patients munch on a sandwich from Au Bon Pain. Because Hanover has long prohibited fast food franchises along its picturesque streets, the hospital quickly became a place for teens to stop for a quick meatball sandwich.[2] A group of "mall rats" even began hanging out at the hospital in the evening, picking up sandwiches from the grocery store and browsing in the bookstore.

The teens were not alone in using the hospital in ways that differed from convention. You can do your banking at the ATM in the small bank branch, drop off your dry cleaning, pick up a video, have your car serviced, and get a haircut while you wait for your doctor or family member. You can make travel arrangements, purchase a gift, and buy flowers. Of course, you could also try on new glasses and fill prescriptions at the pharmacy. A little something for everyone, and a hospital to boot!

Inpatients are separated from the mall, in a quieter, more isolated facility that is still easily accessible to visitors and patients able to use the mall's services. A spiral staircase at the west end of the mall masks the circular in-patient pods. Each pod holds a 36-bed nursing unit, and there are two pods to a floor. The wards were designed to improve nursing efficiency and to give each patient bed a window to the outdoors. The color scheme is soft and restful, and the furniture reminiscent of hotel rooms. Patient rooms, as well as the cafeteria and mall shops, look out upon an evergreen and decid-uous forest that surges into a brilliant array of colors every fall and bursts into bud every spring.

Many other hospitals have been and are being designed using elements of the shopping mall, the hotel, and the home. The functionalism of the post–World War II machine-medicine hospital has given way to brighter, more accessible, patient-centered designs. As architectural writer Mitchel Green has reported, "Designers are emphasizing customer comfort in high-style surroundings, changing designs to encourage family participation, and creating images which evoke an inviting combination of social life and com-munity education."[3] Wood paneling, travertine fireplaces, sculptures, indoor trees, flowers, softer carpeting, and a richer palette of colors greet visitors and draw them through the public areas into the more restrictively designed areas of medical service. Palm trees line the main corridor at the University of California at San Diego's Thornton Hospital. A fantasy atrium sparkles with fairy tale turrets at Cook–Fort Worth's Children's Medical Center. The emergency room waiting area at Miami's Baptist Hospital is filled with overstuffed couches, recessed lighting, and plantings. These new designs ac-centuate accessibility and comfort, deemphasize the ominous nature of med-ical technology, and welcome rather than intimidate patients as they enter the hospital or healthcare facility.

These designs reflect four trends in hospital and healthcare facility ar-chitecture. First, the modernist faith in the hospital has been lost, creating a need for a postmodern approach to designing and managing the hospital. Modernist hospital designers sought essence and unity. Decoration was scrapped, circulation plans simplified, patient rooms standardized, and op-erating rooms sterilized. In small community hospitals, the result was often an easily accessible, easily familiarized place that patients could understand and use. However, in large urban and regional hospitals, especially those that continued to expand, the initial simplicity was lost in growth. Post-modernist architects reject unity as the primary value, seeing the hospital for the fragmented institution it has become. They decorate buildings, insert colors, even soften the facilities' textures and fabrics.[4] In the new, less pragmatic designs, component parts are viewed as separate design issues, the total of which has to work together but not fit together seamlessly.

Second, a more competitive healthcare environment has placed greater emphasis on patients' physical and psychological comfort and the familiarity of the environment. The modern hospital strove for unity through functionalism. Although its sleek corridors were initially easy to navigate, it ultimately failed as a design and as a place to work and be sick. Starkness and sterility proved discomforting and seemed lacking in compassion, when people wanted comfort and care. Architects and designers have borrowed design features from the shopping mall, luxury hotel, and residential home because they soften the hospital's institutional character and simulate spaces that patients and visitors understand and find familiar. Architects also have experimented with brighter light, colorful walls and furnishings, awnings, and other decorative features not previously planned for hospitals. The new hospital retains functionalism while aiming to create a more caring environment.

Third, outpatient medicine has become increasingly important, motivating healthcare providers to decentralize and hospital managers to reconsider the importance of accessibility in the patient's decision to use a particular hospital. The healthcare building boom of the 1990s was in ambulatory, not inpatient, facilities. Significant numbers of hospitals have been closed, forcing some Americans to travel greater and greater distances to receive care. And, as outpatient services have expanded, medicine has increased its reliance on family members to serve as home health providers.

Fourth, hospitals are stressed financially, as insurance and government reimbursements shrink and competition holds down patient co-payments. In some hospitals, this has prompted superficial decoration, which does little to counteract the maze-like corridors and small treatment rooms or mollify patients forced to wait interminably. Some hospitals have opened retail stores inside the hospital building, both to improve the facility's convenience and range of services to its staff, patients, and visitors and to provide another stream of income. While using analogues of hotel and mall implies a commodification of medicine and healthcare, an attempt to make medicine more responsive to consumers, it also potentially damages the precious relationship between patient and provider.

The total effect is a reversal of the century-old philosophy that championed a sterile functionalism and medical purity. As new buildings are constructed, at a rapid pace, scientific elements are being balanced with elements of the older paradigm of care and compassion. Functionalism is still important, but it is defined differently. Peter Whybrow, chairman of UCLA's Department of Neuropsychiatry and Biobehavioral Sciences, had this to say about their redesigned hospital: "Nobody likes going to the hospital anyway, but [we thought] if you had a sense of light and space . . . and could remove some of the onerous sense of doom and dismay that very often surrounds hospitals, [patients] would be much better served."[5] The hope is to return the hospital to its linguistic roots, the Latin *hospes*, serving as host to its guests.

Why the Shopping Mall as Model?

A shopping mall seems an unlikely source of inspiration for hospital design. Few architects and urbanists praise the mall. Although postmodernists are more likely than modernists to favorably view the ordinary environment of the city and suburb, malls have generally been scorned by critics and commentators. While hospitals are perceived as temples where the fundamental questions of life and death are confronted, malls are sites of frivolous entertainment and commerce. Just as medicine is considered a sacred calling, activities at the mall are described in terms of derision and disgust. They are the location of what historian Thomas Bender calls "city lite" and Kenneth Helphand has dubbed "McUrbia."[6] They are, in the minds of some commentators, eyesores that have destroyed downtowns and devastated American public life. Truly an unseemly place to look for a new paradigm.

Yet, both the history of the shopping mall and its current place in American society suggest otherwise. The shopping mall was the outcome of a half-century–long change in urban commercial patterns. It did not just spring out of nowhere to torture downtown department store owners and aggravate the generation gap. Shopping centers and regional malls were the outcome, first, of the suburbanization process that has defined twentieth-century American urbanism. Second, they represent the expansion and deepening of American prosperity and the ability of a broader segment of Americans to join in the consumer culture. And, third, they reflect shifting patterns of commerce, particularly the development of national retail chains and the expansion of consumer credit. The proliferation of automobiles allowed for a faster, more extensive expansion of the city into its fringe. Suburban America became not the margin of urban life but the middle ground between the decaying city and the expanding exurban frontier. Shopping malls challenged, then slew the great downtown department stores, ultimately making their suburban branch stores captives within new malls.

The myth is that America's suburbs were simply bedrooms for people who traveled to the big city to work and shop. However, many suburbs had commercial districts and manufacturing areas from the beginning of their existence. Places such as Panorama City and Westchester (in Los Angeles County) are perfect examples; housing, commerce, and jobs were all coordinated parts of a planned community. However, these were automobile towns. Their commercial districts struggled immediately with parking problems and congestion. As historians Richard Longstreth and Greg Hise have chronicled, in Los Angeles, these mid-century developments led first to the shopping center, then to its big sister the mall.[7] These developments were not aberrations but essential aspects of the new suburban culture.

A shopping center differs from a retail street or marketplace in that it is entirely planned and developed by one owner instead of developing incrementally and consisting of independent stores. The most notable early example was the 1923 Country Club Plaza in Kansas City, developed by J. C. Nichols.[8] Planned as a small group of locally owned stores with an architecturally unified design, managed by one company, and offering off-street parking to serve a larger, upscale residential development in the city's suburbs, Country Club Plaza was immensely successful. It quickly grew to 142 stores, with several parking structures as well as surface parking lots. The success of this shopping center, still going strong today, persuaded developers nationwide to reconsider dependence on downtown shopping and the desirability of urban retail districts, which were uncontrolled and unmanaged, as the traditional mode of commerce in the cities.

The prospect of a more decentralized city, propelled by the growing dependence on the automobile, led innovative architect Victor Gruen to argue in an important 1942 article in *Architectural Record* that shopping centers needed to become community centers. In his plan for the new suburban center, he included not only the typical retail services but also community services such as a library, meeting rooms, and doctors' offices. He recognized that suburbanization diminished the role of the urban center, emphasized life on the fringe, and left a growing number of Americans without a nearby community or civic center. He believed—some say foolishly—that the shopping center could become a downtown for suburbanites.[9]

Gruen's shopping center was only a limited neighborhood amenity, not the mega-mall so familiar today. The latter began in 1956, with the opening of Southdale Shopping Center near Minneapolis.[10] Another Gruen creation, Southdale ushered in the era of the enclosed mall. The stores surrounded a garden court inside a "weather conditioned" building. Southdale attracted public attention not only for its shops but for its sculptured trees and community activities. Able to shop year round in comfort in a place that offered the variety of downtown without the hassle of parking or the uneasiness of downtown life, customers embraced the new shopping mall. During the next decade, thousands of malls were built. Suburban as well as urban commercial areas reeled when confronted with the parking-rich, commercially diverse, easily accessible mall.

The mall became an icon in postwar American life. Generations were initiated in shopping at the mall. Communities did adopt malls as surrogate downtowns, holding civic events and private celebrations there. Senior citizens used the mall as a walking track, and mothers pushed baby carriages and maneuvered children through them. Teenagers became known as "mallrats." Ira Zepp has gone so far as to argue that the shopping mall became America's new ceremonial center.[11] Certainly, the mall became an American institution. For many Americans, the mall is a more familiar space than a city street; they whiz by most streets in their cars, only to act as pedestrians at the mall.

Suburban malls exploited the broad commercial markets created by television advertising, fostering the spread of retail chains and franchises. Instead of local and regional clothing, hardware, or appliance stores, the mall sold national brands. Given the power and pervasive nature of television, those national brands became highly sought after, as well as increasingly the best known products. However, merchandising was only part of

91

the mall's power. In the 1950s, America's cities entered a difficult time, one that was recognized only when the troubles became stark in the 1960s and 1970s. As federal highway, housing, and financial support propelled suburban growth, inner cities decayed. Poverty rates rose, crime rates escalated, and fear spread. The privately owned and controlled malls were perceived as refuges from the city streets. Particularly for a generation of parents worried about their children, the mall seemed a positive alternative, where kids could be safe and entertained.

Parents may have seen malls as safe refuges, but critics viewed them as devilish blotches on the metropolitan landscape. Malls were attacked as artificial, not authentic, as private rather than public, and as commercialized instead of civic spaces. Three generations of urban critics have found the mall wanting. The very characteristics that have made the mall successful are the things that bother critics most. The franchising of American retail has diminished diversity and regional distinctions. The centralizing of stores under one roof has hurt neighborhood businesses and depressed economic development in other parts of the metropolitan area. The functional, enveloping atmosphere of malls is found by many to be oppressive and socially controlled. Still, the mall is accepted, if not loved, as part of the city and the suburb.

The mall's commercialized atmosphere and accessibility became routine components of retail centers. But could such characteristics be applied to the hospital? The key was to apply selective traits. Malls were typically in a suburban location, surrounded by abundant free parking, and conveniently sited for easy access. Once inside a mall, directional signs, both explicit and implicit, guided the shopper through the simple circulation system. Easily read signs and storefronts attracted shoppers, but also ensured that customers knew what services were available and where they might find them. As malls expanded vertically and horizontally, innovative directional guides were installed. A unifying color for carpets and walls distinguished one space from another. Large maps of stores were placed at entrances to inform shoppers of their whereabouts. Hospitals could have the same sense of familiarity and accessibility. They could feel less sterile, more familiar without losing their functionality. Such hopes were ever more relevant in a medical culture where patients were behaving more like clients or customers, doctors were being called providers or caregivers, and medicine was becoming less sacred and more commercial.

MEDICINE MOVES TO THE MALL

A Pluralistic Approach

Of course, not all new hospitals will look like the local mall. Nor will they all employ the mall's pattern for internal traffic circulation, decorative features, parking layout, or enveloping atmosphere. Indeed, some new hospitals will look very different from any shopping mall. Some facilities will be more like homes or hotels, while others will look like nothing else at all. In the new era of hospital design, architects and hospital managers are searching for alternative forms that will allow them to express in their buildings values that modern functionalism could not accommodate. Color, texture, decoration, softness, and difference are atmospheric characteristics that were difficult to fit into the rigid formula of the older hospital. The flexible, pluralistic, postmodern approach allows for greater variety in designs and layouts.

Examples of this variety abound throughout the nation. Wicker furniture sits on terra-cotta flooring in the waiting room of the cancer center at the Baptist Outpatient Center, Jacksonville, Florida. At the Lakeland Medical Center in Austin, Texas, the retention pool appears to flow directly into the atrium lobby. Mummified palm trees line the main corridor of the Thornton Hospital in San Diego, while real deciduous trees grow in Brigham and Women's Hospital atrium in Boston. Arbour Hospital outside Boston looks less like a hospital than a house, with its gables, wood siding, and residential-style windows. The St. Louis Children's Hospital/West County Satellite Center has a terraced and arcaded atrium that contains tables with festive umbrellas and has hanging from its ceiling a hot-air balloon large enough to ride in. For Central Washington Hospital, architects NBBJ of Seattle designed a series of entrance markers in the shape of abstract representations of traditional building components, such as an arch and porte cochere, that are brightly colored to match the fruit grown in the region. The markers provide a new, even controversial, image for the hospital, but they also facilitate patients' navigation through the sprawling complex.[12] The functional cookie-cutter approach to hospital design has been discarded. In public hospitals as well as private ones and general hospitals as well as specialty ones designers have turned to local and regional elements, abstract forms, and atriums.

Such pluralism is emblematic of the broader postmodern movement in architecture. Stephen Verderber and David J. Fine have recently written about the postmodern turn in hospital design. They point out that critics found modern hospital buildings "severe, conservative, monotonous, minimalist, and restrictive." Such critics, borrowing from the work of Robert Venturi, Charles Jenks and other architectural writers, argue that postmodern buildings, conversely, can be "unorthodox in their composition and use of materials, colorful, ironic, ornamental, and historicist." Hospitals are very conservative buildings, administered by cautious boards and symbolic of a staid profession. Not surprisingly, as Verderber and Fine point out, the "giant, centralized medical center was just about the last building type to experience" the influence of postmodernism.[13] Hospital architects turned to analagous public building types, like the shopping mall and hotel, as well as to the home, where architects have been more experimental with color, material, ornament, even irony. These served as models for a generation of architects trying to humanize the hospital.

Patients or Consumers?

A critical component in the process of humanizing the hospital has been a change in the way the patient is viewed. In the new perspective, the patient becomes a consumer of healthcare. Just as retail architecture centered attention on the patron, drawing consumers into the marketplace, hospital architecture is now organized around the values of a consumer culture.[14] As one architectural journal recently noted in describing a new "patient-centered" structure: "Among the happy consequences of [the hospital's] attempt to attract patients . . . is that they are treated like royalty, or at least like hotel guests." Staff members are put through a program emphasizing courtesy and friendliness.[15] Spaces are designed for the convenience of patients, often with the aid of patients.

Whether patients enter through the emergency room, the outpatient clinic, an adjoining medical office building, or the front door, a properly designed facility can serve them as a therapeutic device. These "environments will help ease patient stress, reduce medication levels, and promote shorter hospital stays."[16] At Miami's Baptist Hospital, TRO/The Ritchie Organization reinvented the conventional emergency room by designing "an interior courtyard that continues the Renaissance motifs of the exterior, with brick vaulted ceilings, tile pavers, columns, arches, soft pinks, yellows, and greens."[17] A large skylight shielded by an overhanging oak contributes to a design that evokes the lobby of a hotel rather than the bloody and harried emergency room. And, the hospital's administration has committed to training its staff in "guest relations." The staff at Baptist Hospital attempt to see a patient within five minutes, while liaisons shuttle from exam room to waiting room keeping relatives informed.

A new emphasis on "way-finding" within the hospital diminishes the patient's disorientation upon entering this seldomly frequented space. A consistent complaint of the scientific hospital had been the withholding of information from patients. As one commentator wrote in 1965, "What is it that patients complain of more than anything else in relation to the hospital—'No one told me anything.'"[18] The twentieth-century physician-patient relationship was constructed as a paternalistic relationship, not a collaborative one. This feeling of powerlessness can be reinforced right at patients' entry into the hospital if directions to their destination are unclear. Immediately, they are confused, the last feeling one needs at a time of illness and crisis. The physical environment can soothe or agitate, empower or disempower through the visual clues, sense of place, and image that it extends.

Celebration Health in Orlando, Florida, and St. John's Health Center in Santa Monica, California, represent new or renovated facilities where the entrance has been completely rethought around patients' concerns about getting lost. Many new hospitals emulate mall and hotel entrances, with U-shaped drives leading to a porte cochere since it is both familiar and attractive to patients. Several even go so far as to have valet parking. The driveways of Celebration Health and St. John's are nicely landscaped. When The Ritchie Organization designed a new hospital for Cullman (Alabama) Regional Medical Center, they created an entrance that mimicked a grand southern front porch with a tree-lined walkway. At Sharon (Connecticut) Hospital, Perkins and Will attempted to "reinterpret small-scale New England architecture" by designing an entrance that has a canopy of exposed painted steel, recalling a porte cochere, and leads to a sun-filled corridor, a reminder of a New England porch.[19]

The principle behind these redesigned entry ways has become widely accepted as truth: hospital waiting areas, lobbies, and public spaces in general need to be more accessible, inviting, and easier to find your way through

95

than they were in the past. Such areas may include coffee carts, fast-food restaurants and mall-like shops as well as atriums and sitting areas that could easily pass as hotel lobbies, and the effect makes the hospital less awesome and imposing. As the Rochlin Baran and Balbona design for the Alta Bates Cancer Center in Berkeley, California, suggests, Florence Nightingale's dictum that light is a lifesaver has returned to vogue. The cancer center is located in a basement, so the architects went to elaborate lengths to ensure that light reached deep into the complex. A line of low, canted Mexican limestone piers "thrust their way upward" on the outside, supporting a skylight that brings light into the subterranean public spaces. The result, the architects hope, is a design that is "non-institutional, comfortable, with plenty of light and air."[20] Like Dartmouth-Hitchcock's provision of a window for every inpatient bed, these designs indicate a desire to break through the institutional dreariness of concrete boxes and create a new generation of hospitals.

Inpatients, then, are reaping the benefits of a patient-centered hospital. Too many hospital rooms are still reminders of a sterile past, overcrowded conditions, or simply old hotel closets. And, too many Americans are still unable to gain access to the new hospitals, which are often intended for privately insured clientele. Even with those important limitations, the renewed emphasis on care is affecting all hospital designs, and hopefully more and more medical organizations.

The Patients' Perspective

Throughout the era of the large hospital, commentators have repeatedly blamed inadequacies of the hospital on the refusal of its trustees, managers, and designers to look at the facility from the perspective of the patient. In 1876, as he aided in the design of Johns Hopkins Hospital, John Shaw Billings noted that the literature on hospital construction consisted of hundreds of books, articles, and pamphlets, not one of which was from the patient's perspective. Seventy years later the patient's perspective was still being ignored. When the United States Public Health Service authored a comprehensive series of articles on the architecture of hospitals in 1946, they proudly listed the contribution of "innumerable consultations with doctors, nurses, hospital consultants, dietitians, hospital architects, hospital administrators, technicians, manufacturers" as well as members of their staff. Patients were not listed.[21]

The struggle to maintain the hospital's humanity was recognized almost as soon as scientific medicine started reshaping the institution. In 1918, New York architect William Ludlow published an article calling for "homelike hospitals." In it, he noted a "curious phenomenon," that in designing a "proper environment" for healing in hospitals, architects and physicians had emphasized "negative conditions—no noise, no smells, no ugliness." Such an emphasis was actually a natural outcome of the application of germ theory concepts to living environments. The reasoning was, Germs are everywhere, they are dangerous, so the more sterile the environment, the fewer dangers to the patient. As a result, the oak paneling was pulled off, the rag rugs removed, and the curtains taken down. Patient rooms were painted in institutional colors and furnished to a bare minimum. Ludlow called for "tinted walls," "living plants," and "chintz hangings." The monotony and dreariness of hospitals was already recognized.[22]

In 1960, historian George Rosen noted the contribution of a new voice in shaping the hospital's environment: "As the hospital increased in size and complexity, . . . the organizational relationships within the hospital have been disturbed and have become unstable. It is no longer a question of trustees, administrator, and medical staff alone. Another set of people, the organized consumers, have to be considered and satisfied if possible."[23] As consumers spoke out more and more loudly, hospitals began to incorporate both physical and institutional changes that improved patients' experience of the hospital.

Planetree, a nonprofit group in the San Francisco Bay area, pioneered renovation of the hospital ward. The group was founded by environmentalist and health-care advocate Angelica Thierot, after she had a hospital experience that left her thinking, "Many of the most important moments of people's lives are spent in hospitals. Yet, for the most part, they are the coldest and ugliest places on the earth."[24] She gathered a small group of architects, designers, healthcare professionals, and civic leaders to rethink hospital spaces. In 1985, after a decade of experimentation, the group reached agreement with Pacific Presbyterian Medical Center to renovate a 13-bed nursing unit. The unit was transformed at minimal expense. The central workspace, typically configured to speed the nurse's use of the space, was redesigned to lower physical barriers between nurses and patients, to recreate a relationship between them. In addition, the redesign produced enough space to create a kitchen and lounge for patients and staff. Patient rooms were also subtly altered, with the use of floral sheets and pastel curtains. Plants were encouraged and bulletin boards hung for patients' personal use. In 1986, an architectural writer commented that the older, unrenovated rooms were "unbearably institutional" in comparison to the Planetree ward.

Planetree advocated not only physical but also institutional changes. In the more patient-oriented work spaces, staff reoriented their professional practice. Patients were encouraged to have discussions with doctors and nurses rather than be mute in the presence of authority. Routines were rearranged to cause fewer interruptions of patients' mealtimes and sleep. The kitchen allowed patients and the staff nutritionist to experiment with meals. The overall goal was to reassure patients by allowing them to retain a personal identity, participate in their care, and find comfort in their surroundings.

Reasserting Sentimentality in Labor and Delivery

Perhaps no hospital unit better illustrates the movement to humanize the hospital than the labor and delivery suite. Birth was not a medical procedure for most American women until well into the twentieth century. When pre-eminent hospital architect Edward F. Stevens wrote his influential 1921 book on hospitals, he began his 37-page description of the "maternity department" by noting "a growing call for maternity service in nearly every hospital, whether it be large or small."[25] This call had made necessary the setting apart of a section of the hospital or a new building. This section, he wrote, "should be classed as surgical," which was the viewpoint of most contemporary obstetricians. The "danger of infection" and the "area of open wound" meant that the careful implementation of asepsis was essential.

Maternity units were designed to attract middle- and upper-class women to the hospital while still offering services to those women in need of charity care. Stevens described a variety of bedding accommodations, but most units had wards and private rooms. The wards ranged from 2 beds (what would acquire the name "semiprivate room" in the 1950s) to 16 beds. He anticipated that wealthier women would come to the hospital for a few days before and after the birth. Poorer women, he wrote, "frequently enter from one to three months before confinement. Such women assist about the hospital work and in a measure repay for their care when sick." In most hospitals, private room patients shared the labor and delivery rooms with the ward patients. However, at St. Luke's Hospital in New Bedford, Massachusetts, even these were separated. St. Luke's had three delivery rooms, one each for private, semiprivate, and ward patients.

When Isadore Rosenfield considered maternity and pediatric departments in 1947, he began by noting the extraordinary rise of hospital births during the twentieth century. While only 33.6 percent of live births occurred in hospitals in 1933, 76 percent did in 1943. The maternity department had become an accepted part of hospital life. Rosenfield focused most attention on the nursery, with barely a mention of the delivery and recovery rooms. Babies were expected to spend roughly 10 days in the hospital, down from 14 in the 1930s. Too many nurseries were "cheerless and hazardous locations" where "infants are herded together one bassinet against the other without any separation between them."[26] Further, they were separated from their mothers by long corridors, "which are public streets so far as their bacteria laden nature is concerned." The preoccupation continued to be with fighting potential illness, not with nurturing relationships between child and mother, father, and other family.

Birth was medicalized in the scientific hospital at the insistence of mostly male obstetricians, who first encouraged their patients to enter the hospital, then dictated the rules of their care. For instance, in October 1964, Dr. John Morton said in argument against allowing fathers into the delivery room: "The day we are born is the most dangerous one of our lives, and everyone in the delivery room must have a definite duty. . . . *This room is no place for sentimentality, sightseeing, sex gratification, or salesmanship.* Historically many minor deities have presided over obstetrical rites. We believe in a strictly professional approach." Fathers had no place in this medical space because (1) it is too emotional a time for them and (2) the mother is "simply not at her romantic best in a delivery room."[27] California outlawed the presence of fathers in delivery rooms for just these reasons.

In the past four decades, maternity rooms have become the most domesticated spaces in the hospital. Architect Roslyn Lindheim, who was a central Planetree figure, stated that the "alternative birth center represents an attempt to duplicate the amenities of a home within the technological environment of the hospital." Hospitals eager to have maternity cases, and the pediatric clients they produce, compete to provide mothers the best spaces, the most attention, and the least-institutional experience possible. As architects Richard Miller and Earl Swensson relate about the North Florida Women's Center, "The prevailing look is noninstitutional, with residential-style furnishings, ample natural light, and extensive outdoor landscaping." The center includes a woman's resource center, health and fitness center, ambulatory surgical facilities, and labor and delivery rooms that are "residential in decor" and overlook a lake.

At Baptist Hospital in Miami, the new Lake Pavilion/Family Birth Center is a separate structure on a rapidly expanding medical campus.[28] The 50,000-square-foot center represents the nationwide trend to domesticate hospital birth and to separate outpatients and birthing mothers from more seriously ill inpatients. The Ritchie Organization designed a space that dispersed activity by creating "intimate clusters" with a "relaxed, nonclinical setting." The maternity suite's eight rooms include such homelike furnishings as armoire-like cabinets containing a television, music recordings, and a little refrigerator; oversize sleeper chairs; and "of course—rocking chairs." The rooms look out on courtyards or lakes, reflecting another general trend— to calm patients through connection with the attractive views outside.

The new maternity rooms at Baptist Hospital have served as a model for the hospital's customer service. Numerous writers have suggested ways to reorient hospital staff, improve patients' experience by altering the organizational assumptions of most hospital care. Healthcare consultant Chuck Musfeldt wrote in *Hospitals* in 1992, that he had found ten key attributes of the "hassle-free" hospital. They ranged from such social issues as "everyone treats everyone else as a customer" and "nurses learn the names of patients' families and visitors," to organizational concerns such as "radiology and lab reports get onto the chart in a timely manner" and "patients receive a daily schedule of what's going to happen to them." At Tallahassee (Florida) Memorial Regional Medical Center, as reported in *Hospitals* in 1992, CEO Duncan Moore instituted a strategic plan that emphasized customer service and a satisfying practice environment, believing that the two are synergistic, not opposite. Units were encouraged to identify their missions, current conditions, and a vision. Employees were encouraged to imagine themselves less as employees working for other employees and more as "doing the work for the patient."

The ultimate goal, as has become clear in the literature over the 1990s, is to construct such wonderful spaces staffed by such competent and caring people that, in the words of *Business Week*, the result is "hospitals you may hate to leave." The *Business Week* article reported on the small number of upper-end private hospitals where "free newspapers, private bathrooms, and refrigerators are common amenities." A growing number of hospitals have staffed concierge desks that serve as visitor information centers. In each case, from the earliest discussion of patient-centered medicine, the purpose of these design changes has been to give patients/customers/clients more control over their hospital experience. As patient Patricia York described the feeling, after five days in the deluxe unit at Michael Resse Hospital in Chicago, "When you go into a hospital, you lose control of your life. It's nice to have surroundings that give you your dignity back."[29] These redesigned spaces create that feeling of greater control by mimicking places that patients find more familiar than the hospital. In homelike maternity rooms, hotel-like lobbies and mall-like traffic circulation systems, it is hoped, patients will feel more welcome and more able to navigate, even as they confront the fears that accompany any serious medical event.

Of course, whether the control is real or an illusion depends on more than fresh flowers or easily decipherable signs, and an important question is whether the hospital's institutional life has shifted as fast or far as its design has.

The Changing Meaning of *Outpatient*

As patient-centeredness is shaping space and practice within inpatient facilities, changing medical practice and fiscal conditions are driving the development of bigger, more accessible, less frightening ambulatory care centers. Hospitals are increasingly becoming critical care facilities, with other types of care "unbundled" and moved from the hospital into convalescent homes, hospices, even hotel-style recovery units. Ambulatory care is a prime example. Brigham and Women's Hospital in Boston, St. Luke's Medical Center in Milwaukee, and Scripps Memorial Hospital in San Diego are just

a few hospitals that during the 1990s have constructed new facilities to accommodate their outpatients. Constructing separate outpatient units has
become popular because ambulatory care facilities can be built and maintained for less expense than hospitals, they segregate outpatients from inpatients, and they offer another way for a hospital or HMO to differentiate the
care it offers from that of competitors. The designs of these outpatient facilities are often bolder and more dramatic than those of inpatient spaces
but, like the new designs of hospital rooms, are intended to make the clinic
a more comforting place.[30]

What a change from earlier in the century. Then, few organized health
services for ambulatory care existed. The vast majority of the non-poor went
to a physician's private office, not to a hospital. Or, the doctor visited them,
when they contracted measles or mumps. Poor people depended on either
charitable care provided by physicians or upon themselves and their families. Some, fortunate enough to live in New York or a few other large cities,
stopped by their local dispensary. The dispensary had originated in the eighteenth century in England and was quickly brought to America.[31] Dispensaries were founded in Philadelphia, New York, and Boston around the time
of the Revolution. The idea spread slowly. However, by 1890 more than 130
dispensaries had been established in the Atlantic Coast states, the vast majority of them in the few large American cities. They offered services free or
at minimal cost to those unable to afford their own physicians. And, they
were very busy. As early as 1860, New York's dispensaries treated more than
130,000 patients, and the number rose to almost 900,000 by 1900.

Dispensaries were linked historically to the development of early efforts
to implement a broad-based public health system. Physicians treated people
who came to dispensaries or went out to people who could not travel. Later,
in New York, legendary public health physician Stephen Smith organized a
sanitary survey that depended on dispensary physicians to report on the
city's conditions. Given that stockyards still stood adjacent to schools, the
picture was none too flattering. By the beginning of the twentieth century,
the dispensary, joined by hospital outpatient departments and specialty hospital clinics, offered a wide variety of ambulatory clinics. Health policy expert Michael M. Davis reported on almost 6,000 such places in the United
States in 1922. Roughly 22 percent of them were housed in hospitals, a per-
centage that would grow dramatically over the succeeding decades.

Davis realized that the dispensaries could not compete with hospital outpatient clinics. He illustrated this fact in a graphic woodcut titled "The Clinic Tree." The "Old Style Dispensary" is shown as a short, bare branch of the tree, while "Hospital O-P-D," "TB," "Specialties," and others are flowering branches. Many of the same reasons that motivated physicians to move their patients from home to hospital inpatient beds influenced the success of outpatient departments. Edward Stevens summed up these causes when he wrote about where the outpatient department should be located. The department's "entrance should be as accessible as possible from the main streets, and yet not be so placed as to interfere with ambulances, automobiles, patients, or visitors coming to the building." Outpatient medicine, he implied, was different from the primary hospital mission, so it should be physically separated from it. However, clinics should be accessible to "the laboratories of the hospital and the X-ray department." Once again, just as the hospital's technology had provided it with a competitive edge over home and physician's office for inpatients, they provided cause for directing outpatients to hospitals.[32]

The design of rooms in the outpatient department, Stevens declared, should be flexible, so that the various types of clinics could be housed in the same rooms on different nights. Charles Rosenberg makes the point that outpatient clinics and dispensaries played an important role in specialty clinical training. During a week or over two weeks, outpatients might in the same building see specialists in surgery, venereal diseases, eye-ear-nose-and-throat problems, orthopedics, gynecology, and dentistry. Outpatient departments served as a prime place for young physicians to see a wide variety of disorders. The waiting rooms would be jammed, because patients paid nothing or very little, and they were one way of holding down rising medical expenses, as well as of getting second opinions relatively cheaply. Particularly popular clinics were those for the children, many of whom had orthopedic or respiratory problems.[33]

It was in outpatient departments that social service departments in hospitals developed. The first was opened in Boston in 1905. Here, social workers collaborated with clinicians to improve medical outcomes. The social service department seems a logical extension of the Progressive Era concern about public and community health, typified by many settlement houses, visiting nursing services, and other attempts to improve individuals' and group's health. Significantly, Stevens suggests that the social service office "should be easily accessible from the out-patient department. . . ." Through social service intervention, patients could be screened economically, and follow-through could improve compliance with medical treatments.

The early outpatient clinics reflected the economic and social divisions that continued to influence the physical spaces of healthcare. Throughout descriptions of such clinics, their charitable beneficence is repeatedly noted. Illustrations show outpatient departments that were often dark, crowded spaces where people appear to have waited long times for their care. The tired faces of the people seated in hard-backed chairs leave the same impression as those of patients who must wait for hours in today's public hospitals. In addition, outpatient clinics were the only places that African Americans could receive care at some southern hospitals. Even there, they were segregated. Stevens reproduces the plan of Macon (Georgia) City Hospital. While the five treatment rooms are not distinguished by race, two waiting rooms—the larger for "colored"—are clearly demarcated, along with accompanying restrooms.[34]

As late as the 1940s, outpatient departments were expected to serve largely or exclusively charity patients, those unable to afford the full inpatient expense. Such departments were typical only in urban hospitals, and even there they were not always included. Architect Charles Neergaard recorded in a 1939 discussion of small hospitals that of "the five general divisions [of a hospital]. . . , the Outpatient Department is occasionally omitted." He noted, though, that such omissions were quickly becoming past fashion, since "with increasing development of social consciousness and recognition of social needs, facilities for outpatients are being incorporated in more and more hospitals." Even so, seven years later, E. H. L. Corwin reported that studies showed that only 5 percent of cities with a population less than 100,000 had an outpatient department.[35]

The 1950 design of St. Clare's Hospital, Schenectady, New York, by York and Sawyer, Architects, suggests the continuing peripheral nature of outpatients to this small community hospital. The outpatient department was located in the west wing, next to the emergency room. While the connection of emergency rooms and outpatient departments was quite typical, at St. Clare's it presented a particular problem. Any patient admitted into the hospital from the emergency room would have to pass through the outpatient waiting room on a stretcher. Although the architects were concerned, they argued, "It is a functional arrangement which is difficult to avoid unless something else more serious be sacrificed to obtain another grade entrance, which in this case was impossible."[36] Apparently, wheeling a seriously ill patient through other waiting patients was not as serious an issue as one might think. The race and class of the people who would be sitting there might have played some role in the architects willingness to accept such a flaw.

Just as hospitals were originally for the poor then attracted other Americans, the outpatient service went through a transition from being almost exclusively a charity affair to being an integral part of the private healthcare system. The transition appears to have happened between the 1940s and the 1960s, with the change occurring incrementally. Several articles in 1965 on the meaning of *outpatient* suggest that the transition was well under way. Medical scholar Jerry Alan Solon called *outpatient care* "a term in search of a concept." While recognizing that "outpatient care is entering a new and dynamic phase," Solon asked if the distinctions between outpatient, inpatient, and home care might actually be arbitrary and provide an obstacle to integrating care no matter where and when it occurred.[37]

The obstacles to such comprehensive care, he recognized, were considerable. Physicians preferred to retain patients within their private practice, seeing them at home or in their offices. Hospitals organized their services around hospital admissions versus outpatient visits. Further, *outpatient* remained tainted in many middle class minds, as referring to charitable care. As Solon wrote, "The origins and traditions of the hospital outpatient have imbued the term 'outpatient' with connotations of charity and indigence, inducing a quest for a more dignifying term." *Ambulatory care* was favored by a growing number of hospitals, because it "apparently accords dignity at the same time that it seemingly characterizes the type of service." Solon disagreed, arguing that *ambulatory care* actually confused the situation, by putting even greater emphasis on the patient's ability to walk, which for many outpatients was simply not true.

The expansion of ambulatory care, especially within hospitals, has been extensive. Inpatient hospital admissions, hospital occupancy rates, and the average length of a patient's stay have all been declining since at least 1981, and the number of outpatient visits has skyrocketed. In 1965, approximately

125 million outpatients visited American Hospital Association–registered hospitals. By 1985, the number had risen to 282 million. By 1995, it had grown to 483 million.[38] Clearly, outpatients had become a prime source for hospital service and reimbursement.

Even as hospitals are forced to close because of the declining number of inpatients, new ambulatory care buildings have been opened and old ones expanded, redesigned, and expanded again to meet the growing numbers. According to the F. W. Dodge division of the McGraw-Hill Companies, between 1992 and 1996, hospital construction contract awards declined from $6.8 billion to $5.3 billion. During the same period, contracts for neighborhood care centers, specialty clinics, nursing homes, and other such facilities rose from $4.1 billion to $5.6 billion, or from 39.8 million square feet of building construction to nearly 53 million.[39] Outpatient care is no longer the stepchild of the hospital's "real" work, it is a battleground where patients are attracted to the comprehensive services (other primary and specialty care, and in some cases convalescent and hospice care) offered by that hospital, or chain of hospitals, or HMO system. The buildings are more welcoming, engaging, comfortable, accessible, and even diverse because they have taken on such an importance to the overall success of the institution.

Those changes are manifested in the ambulatory clinics and buildings being constructed around the nation. The buildings articulate a new direction in healthcare design through their entrances and lobbies, comfortable patient waiting rooms, softer, warmer colors, and use of decoration and ornamentation. Interior designer Jain Malkin has argued that the two challenges of the 1990s have been "creating healing environments" and learning "how to design for specific patient populations."[40] The hospital is no longer a unitary place, it is now a "village" of spaces, with each taking its own character from the needs of its patient population. Ambulatory medicine is shaped by the repeated visits of primarily chronically ill people. The buildings do not have to be constructed to the same building codes as inpatient hospital spaces, nor should they be, given the heightened need for easy access and patient's sense of control.

Just as in hospital inpatient spaces, redesigned lobbies have been used to redefine the the atmosphere. The lobby serves as the door to the patient's experience of the space. As noted above, previously the door to outpatient services might well be obscure, might force patients to pass through spaces where they were uncomfortable, and leave them marginalized. At St. Luke's Medical Center in Milwaukee, Wisconsin, Bobrow/Thomas and Associates reconfigured an obscured entrance to ease patients entry to the building while directing them to the appropriate area.[41] The new seven-story, 165,000-square-foot outpatient wing was designed to draw light into the main lobby and the two-story galleria that forms its circulation spine. The galleria is punctuated with skylights that are used to help define the various departments along the spine. The lobby, with its curving cherry wood wall, becomes an easily identified landmark that helps orient visitors, guides patients, and signals a comfortable professionalism as the building's identity.

As lobbies have become grander and more expressive, designers have increasingly introduced atriums into hospitals. For instance, Boston's Brigham and Women's Hospital constructed a new building to consolidate their scattered ambulatory care services. The building's 300-foot atrium has become its defining feature. Older outpatient spaces were tucked away in the basement or back of the building, but this atrium eases access through the use of powerful directional design. Elevators are prominently displayed and, unlike in so many older hospitals, corridors are well defined. The atrium, though, is important for more than its functional qualities. As a leading hospital interior designer, Jain Malkin states, "The atrium succeeds magnificently. . . . The scale of the space, with its focus on coffers and skylights, lifts the spirit. The complexity and intricacy of forms and patterns, and layering of materials make the space visually stimulating. Every surface . . . is carefully considered in terms of proportion, texture, and color."[42] Sitting or walking through the atrium, one feels in control, not caught in a maze.

Commercial spaces have long used atriums, in either lobbies or indoor courtyards, as relief from narrow corridors and windowless spaces. At Westside Pavilion shopping mall in Los Angeles, architect Jon Jerde constructed an arcade atrium that spans more than half the mall. The steel-and-glass peaked ceiling brings valuable light into the building, and the sunlight plays on the multiple stairways and escalators. Of course, atriums became almost mandatory in luxury hotels built in the 1980s and early 1990s. In a John Portman hotel, the atrium became the interior space. Atriums are larger-than-life spaces, so to speak, giving buildings a grandeur and majesty.

Majesty, though, can be as intimidating as sterility. The new hospital spaces must not only alter the patient's perception of the hospital; they must also greet them warmly. The earlier highly functional, sleek lobbies introduced patients to the busy medical workplace. Designs that resonate of home, hotel, and mall send different messages—of comfort, familiarity, and power sharing between patient and provider. At Sharon Hospital in Connecticut, Perkins and Will architects designed the corridor waiting area as "a reminder of the ubiquitous New England porch" and the two-story lobby as an allusion to the old family parlor.[43] The Cleveland Clinic's large (620,000 sq. ft.) ambulatory services building, which accommodates 22 clinics in a 14-story granite and glass structure, is planned to offer views of the campus green from waiting rooms. The green is a constant in the continually shifting world of patients as they move through space from waiting to treatment, treatment to diagnostic test, test to treatment, treatment to billing and appointments.

The natural elements are one way to soothe; warm colors and soft fabrics are another. When Horton Plaza, designed by Jon Jerde, opened in San Diego in 1985, people were startled by the rich palette that he had chosen for a shopping mall. His choices alluded to the vibrant colors used south of the nearby Mexican border, but they also announced the special nature of shopping at this inner-city mall located in an urban redevelopment area. Jerde's creation resembled a village of tiered stores gathered around narrow passageways. Horton Plaza's vibrancy contrasts sharply with the look of most hospitals. Muted earth colors might greet you in the lobby, but institutional colors, mostly white and more white, covered the rest. Using white paint on walls replaced whitewashing walls, which was one way of cleansing them in nineteenth-century hospitals, but the effect was the same. White walls were not distracting to surgeons and others embarked on scientific and medical exploration. White walls were simple, in keeping with the functional approach. White walls symbolized cleanliness.

Various writers argued against the whitening of the hospital. Architect William Ludlow expressed his hopes in 1921 when he wrote, "I am entirely convinced that we shall commonly see the hospital of the near future with tinted walls, with interesting but simple stencil on ceilings and at angles, with living plants here and there, pictures . . . set flush with the walls and glassed over, arranged perhaps so that they may be changed occasionally, and even—shocking to the thought of tradition—plain washable chintz hangings of quaint design and appropriate color to break the plainness which the weary eye everlastingly roams over."[44] While it it has taken longer than he hoped, the wait is over. Even as some designers and managers worry about diminishing the seriousness of the medical mission, they have reapplied the color and texture common in earlier hospital spaces. Again, ambulatory care buildings and clinics have been leaders in this regard. Jain Malkin displays a remarkable variety of colors and textures in her book on hospital interior design.

Specialty Centers

As the number of treatments available through outpatient care has expanded, an increasing number of patients under the care of specialists are outpatients. Specialty facilities, ranging from cancer centers to children's hospitals, are being constructed to serve these patients. In these facilities, as well as in general ambulatory clinics, accessibility, comfort, and familiarity play an important role in the design. Susan Doubilet wrote in *Progressive Architecture* in 1986 about the H. Lee Moffitt Cancer Center that designers had worked hard—perhaps too hard in this case—to make entrances, signs, and spaces look "normal," so that patients would be comforted.[45]

Children's hospitals may be the best example of specialty facilities that are trying to soothe their patients through design. David Schwarz's Cook–Fort Worth Children's Hospital is a prime example. In joining two hospitals, Schwarz had the challenge, and the opportunity, to create new, dramatic spaces. The atrium is walled with "lavishly embellished fairy-tale 'buildings' fashioned of drywall and imagination."[46] The intent is to blend access and relaxation, creating enchanting spaces that comfort staff and engage children and visitors. Even the parking lot is a confection of a castle, with turrets and an illusionary drawbridge entrance, all concocted for a few thousand dollars. And, children are carried through these spaces not in old-fashioned wheelchairs but in little red wagons.

Such elaborate designs raise the so-far unanswered question of whether the hospital environment can help heal? Such groups as the Center for Healthcare Design and the American Architectural Foundation (AAF) are funding or publicizing studies that suggest a connection between an amiable environment and faster healing, or at least better psychological attitudes while ill. The AAF's web page relates the feelings of one father about his

HUMANIZING THE HOSPITAL

five-year-old's experience at the Louise Salter Packard Children's Hospital at Stanford University Hospital: "The building itself is wonderful. I did not realize before this how much architecture could raise the human spirit." Providing daybeds for parents, ample spaces for children's toys, and allowing patients to at least slightly individualize their own space, the hospital is taking the approach that "when you hospitalize a child, you hospitalize the family."[47] Still, tying good design to improved health is hard.

Medical Malls

Modern hospitals have long been more than one simple building with one task. They have incorporated inpatient care centers, outpatient care clinics, laboratories, research facilities, even, increasingly, convalescent and terminal care facilities. Architectural and interior designers have responded to the hospital's dynamic nature and the unbundling of services into separate spaces by imagining the hospital as an assemblage rather than the unified multistory block common during the mid-twentieth century. The shopping mall again provides a pertinent model. The mall ties together the individual stores through a circulation spine and by creating a common place. The designers of Dartmouth-Hitchcock used the mall as a unifying feature to connect and combine inpatient, outpatient, research, and educational elements. At the Cleveland Clinic, an outdoor mall binds together the large, numerous buildings by serving as a constant reference for staff, patients, and visitors. Other hospitals have embraced the mall as the generic design for bundling together their disparate pieces. They have literally created the medical center as mall.

The "medical mall" was pioneered in Texas in 1974 when Robert Wright opened Medical City Dallas. Medical City was a 1.56 million-square-foot medical and retail mixed development. The complex housed traditional medical facilities, such as an emergency room, outpatient clinic, and inpatient hospital, as well as three medical office towers with 130 physicians' offices, a play area for children, two pharmacies, and 21 nonmedical businesses. These other businesses included a gourmet food shop, a bank, six restaurants, a travel agency, clothing store, hair salon, and two newsstands. In the original design, the elements were oriented around a single atrium, from which the various services radiated. As the complex expanded, new atriums were added, connected to the original by concourses. One patient's wife declared, "If you have to be in a hospital, this is certainly the place to be."[48] In the 1970s, few hospital complexes emulated Medical City, but as market competition escalated and ambulatory care (including outpatient surgery) became more important in the 1980s, the hospital as mall became more sensible.

Advertising executive Jane Boone wrote that Medical City Dallas had served as a prototype for facilities in Austin and Fort Worth, Texas, because the mall helped organize the wide range of medical services into a comprehensible configuration for consumers. In this sense, medical malls are cousins to their retail relatives. Healthcare consumers are not going to impulsively stop by the medical mall looking for a surgery sale; however, if a person visiting a relative in the inpatient facility is guided through a central atrium in which signs announce flu shots, free mammograms, or new dental services, they may plan for another trip to the complex for that purpose, or they may impulsively act to get that flu shot. If such promotions are reinforced by the presence of a pharmacy, optician, and fast-food franchise, the medical mall then offers consumers a wide range of services that may make them feel more comfortable with using medical services. The mall becomes a means of not only selling services, but also gaining loyalty from consumers faced with a wide range of competitive resources.[49]

In the late 1980s and early 1990s, medical malls sprouted up around the country. St. John's Regional Medical Center in Oxnard, California, developed a mall between the existing hospital and professional building that combines ambulatory services with retail activities. At Winchester (Virginia) Medical Center the mall is used as Dartmouth-Hitchcock's is, as a spine tying together a variety of hospital-based medical services. Each service has a separate entrance and the entire mall is oriented around a landscaped courtyard.[50] Other medical institutions viewed the mall as a means of bringing together a disparate group of healthcare services. The Jackson (Mississippi) Medical Mall hoped to attract a local clinic, the health department, and a comprehensive health center. Public and private organizations grouped together to create a medical center for the convenience of the public.[51] Medical practitioners would be joined by retail stores, including a bank, pharmacy, clothing store, dry cleaner, and restaurants.

In one case, a retail mall became a hospital. In a Houston, Texas, suburb, Kingwood Hospital was opened in a failed shopping mall. A $40 million project renovated the former Deauville Mall, using approximately two-thirds of the building for a community hospital that offers 120 acute-care beds, a sports medicine center, physical rehabilitation center, and psychiatric outpatient facility. Behind the hospital in the same building runs a medical retail corridor that hospital administrators hope will include a day care center, eye clinic, home health center, and various health-related retail services. The developers of the for-profit hospital added skylights and upgraded the planting intended for the mall so as to attract well-insured patients to the hospital's services.[52]

The line between hospital and mall is continually blurring. As ambulatory clinics and surgical centers open in mini-malls, neighborhood shopping centers, and even in regional malls, and as architects look to hotels and malls as models for hospital spaces, the expected visual boundaries collapse. Taking a look at the central corridor of Bronson Methodist Hospital in Kalamazoo, Michigan, one wonders, "Is it a shopping mall? Is it a hospital?"

Cosmetic Surgery or Revolutionary Change?

While contemporary architects have worked diligently to make the hospital more hospitable, they have also been made aware of the intensely competitive aspects of the medical marketplace. Hospitals must draw patients (customers) if they are to succeed in this environment. Architects have been enlisted in this effort. "The patient/customer now shops for cost, quality, and convenience in healthcare services," writes one hospital architect. "Responding to this new marketplace, hospitals of the future will transform themselves into a resemblance of successful commercial and retail centers."[53] He continues:

> The new age health center will be the connecting point for a variety of different services including laser clinics, regeneration centers, biotech research, birthing centers, hospice and self-care. Patients, staff, and equipment will shuttle between buildings and over parking lots on Disneyesque skywalks. Convenient self-service medical malls will encourage out-of-pocket spending for a wide array of ambulatory care services at health shops, discount pharmacies, and wellness programs. These new health cen-

ters will adopt standard features from the airline and hotel industries, introducing computerized, curbside admitting services and building inpatient towers around large greenhouse atrium spaces.

In a strategy reminiscent of the early-nineteenth-century hospital designs that emulated civic buildings to gain credibility with urban residents, new hospital designs mimic retail and resort buildings to gain the trust of savvy health and medical consumers.

Such a merging of medicine and the market is symbolized in Florida Hospital's Celebration Health in central Florida. Entertainment giant Disney has joined with the Seventh-day Adventist Church's Florida Hospital to develop a comprehensive healthcare center that includes a diagnostic imaging center, a wellness center, an ambulatory surgery facility, and a sports medicine facility in addition to a 60-bed inpatient facility. The hospital opened in 1997, part of the larger planned community, which boasts neotraditional urban plans intended to construct a community environment for the roughly 20,000 residents. The health prevention goals of the medical center are integrally related to the overall aims of the community named Celebration to create a modern subdivision that reflects mid-twentieth-century community values and services.

Celebration Health tries to be as welcoming as possible. Four rows of palm trees grace its U-shaped entrance. The Spanish-style design has almost wall-length windows, bringing light into the hotel-like atrium lobby. As at Thornton Hospital in La Jolla, California, the medical services are not visible immediately upon entering the building; they are sheltered off the main corridor. The hospital is divided spatially and institutionally into a series of centers: diabetes, dental, imaging, fitness, rehabilitation and sports medicine, and education, among others. Florida Hospital is committed to providing comprehensive healthcare rather than conventional medical care to its "guests." The Women's Center, for instance, provides standard services, such as obstetrics and gynecology and mammograms, but it also offers spa services and nutritional counseling. The delivery rooms are, to quote the hospital's promotional materials, "bright, spacious, home-like suites, complete with televisions, VCRs, and a sleeper sofa for Dad." In the competitive Florida healthcare market, the last generation's reforms have become part of daily business.

However, as Lucette Lagnado has noted in a *Wall Street Journal* article, the hospital is actually a compromise in the tension between "the wellness people" and the "doctors."[54] These two poles of the debate about the future of healthcare envision the future as a place, on the one hand, without hospitals or, on the other, with an ever greater need for hospitals. Celebration Health's executives refused to side with either vision, arguing that, the "hospital of the future has to speak two languages—the language of health and wellness and the language of healing, which is curing disease." Physically, in the words of one executive, the "Street of Health," the front corridor off which the various medical centers and retail entities radiate, coexists with the "Corridor of Healing," the inpatient facility "with its beds and sick people in gowns." In both places the patient is supposed to come first, and the mind-set of functional medicine, which sometimes treated patients as disembodied organs, has been banished.

Making it all work, though, is hard. Healthcare designer Barbara J. Huelat reports that when she went to Celebration Health as a patient, she encountered some the problems traditionally associated with hospitals. She waited a long time, in a "drab seclusion room . . . know[ing] that we were surrounded by glorious but inaccessible design." She was "impressed" by the waiting room for the emergency room, as well as the courtesy and helpfulness of the staff. Celebration Health had, in her words, "the character of a health spa, not a hospital. It is easy to navigate. We saw none of the institutional carts lining the halls, or negative medical smells." Still, inside the emergency room, beyond the waiting room, which "would put most hotel lobbies to shame," the same issues of patient's lack of control and level of discomfort once again arose.[55]

Celebration Health was intended to be an innovative place influenced by a wide range of expert opinion from around the nation. Other hospitals may not be so committed to changing both space and place. The highly charged nature of the healthcare market makes one skeptical of hospital managers' motives when new glitzy buildings are constructed or older units renovated. Pressured to compete with nearby hospitals, watching rebellious physicians open their own ambulatory surgicenters and giant healthcare systems gobble up hospitals nationwide, managers constantly need to be coming up with ways to maintain their current patient base as well as attract the new business that allows an institution to continue to grow. Most managers focus their concerns on cost, but those that wish to attract wealthy and middle-class Americans are realizing that ambiance plays a role in maintaining consumer loyalty in a competitive market. Will the changes stop at cosmetic alterations intended to keep that market satisfied, or will the changes affect medical practice as well as the spaces in which it occurs?

In too many designs, the changes stop at the entrance, with its atrium lobby, new furniture, and wood paneling. The interior medical spaces are left untouched, often disassembling into a maze of small rooms with few directional guides and a lack of concern for the patient's comfort. Hospitals continue to struggle with their dynamic nature. The expansion of ambulatory services, whether surgical, primary care, or specialized, or simply the addition of more patients, has the same effect as in the old expansionary period of inpatient services: the space is constantly under pressure to hold more people and to perform more tasks than what it was originally designed to do. Patients wait a long time, are squeezed into small evaluation rooms, and are sent home to minister to themselves, because of a lack of inpatient space or limits to insurance reimbursement. The pressures are not abating. As Wanda F. Jones, a healthcare consultant, argues, "The pace of change in the healthcare industry will only get faster in the next few years."[56] Jones and most others keeping an eye on these changes view ambulatory care as the area where the greatest growth and strain will occur.

A consumer orientation to healthcare and hospital design inevitably reflects the broader commodification of healthcare that has characterized the economy of medical services since the mid-1970s. In the postmodern medical world, doctors have been redefined as providers, patients are customers purchasing "product lines" that have been rigorously evaluated through statistical techniques not only for their medical effectiveness but for customer satisfaction as well. "Product lines" must reap profits to gain a place in the medical market. The hospital, broadly construed, has become the commercial site for such transactions.

As this new consumerist aesthetic has emerged, it makes sense to inquire about its historical implications and significance. In part, no doubt, it reflects a responsiveness to an ongoing critique of medical authority and paternalism in the doctor-patient relationship and new desires to "empower" patients. The development of new, user-friendly hospitals that seem neither imposing nor threatening is clearly an unobjectionable development.

Nonetheless, these buildings do not reflect a deeper critique, that of the biomedical paradigm, which has dominated Western medicine since the turn of the century. Nor do they offer alternative visions of disease causality, risk, or responsibility.

The new hospital architecture is an explicit attempt to "civilize the machine."[57] And while it reflects a respect for patient comfort, more significantly it reflects the further commodification of healthcare within the contemporary market of healthcare services. The hospitals built in the past three decades were designed to compete for patients in a shrinking and intensely competitive market. And not just any patient; they seek to draw paying patients, the well-insured and those willing to pay for additional services out of pocket. In the explicit desire to obfuscate the architectural boundaries between the resort hotel, the shopping mall, and the hospital is a powerful implicit message that medicine is a business, medical care is a commodity. This is not a new development, but only recently has it enlisted the powerful symbolic logic of architecture. Reading the architecture of this complicated machine offers insights into medical theory and practice and the nature of the medical economy and culture. The history of the logic and aesthetic of hospital construction reveals core medical values and ideals and also broader cultural notions of disease, health, and healthcare.

Mini-Mall Medicine

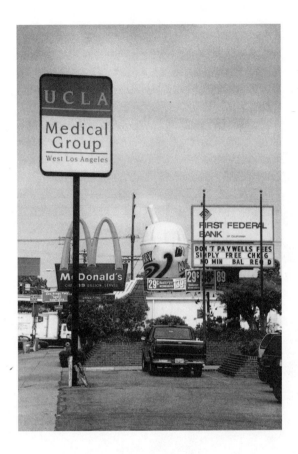

Los Angeles, 1999. In the new healthcare landscape, where medical facilities vie with all kinds of commercial establishments for the consumer's attention, the professional office's sign must be as bold as its neighbors'. *Photograph by Beverlie Conant Sloane.*

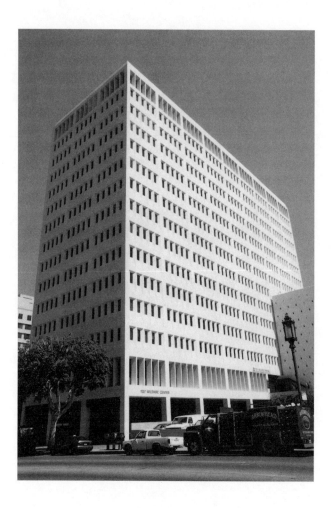

Los Angeles, ca. 1964. In post–World War II America, physicians congregated in sleek modernist office buildings like the Wilshire Metropolitan Medical Center, whose design signaled their separation from the tumult of the marketplace. *Photograph (2000) by Beverlie Conant Sloane.*

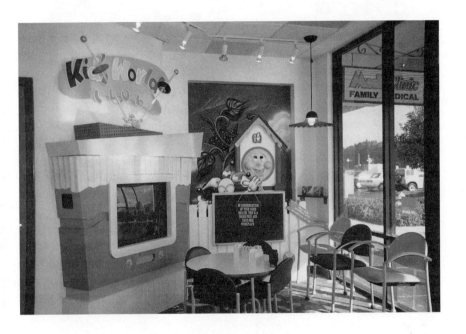

Orlando, Florida, 1990s. Medi-Clinic, a family medicine clinic operated by Main Street Physicians in a strip mall near Disney's Celebration community, has a bright and playful waiting area that echoes its larger neighbor's philosophy of humanizing the residential urban environment. *Photograph by Beverlie Conant Sloane.*

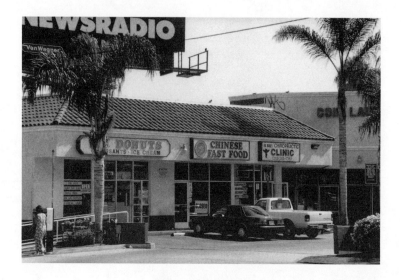

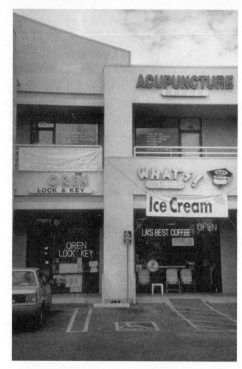

Los Angeles, 1990s. Alternative and complementary medical services are found throughout Los Angeles, tucked into small strip malls and mini-malls. *Photographs by Beverlie Conant Sloane.*

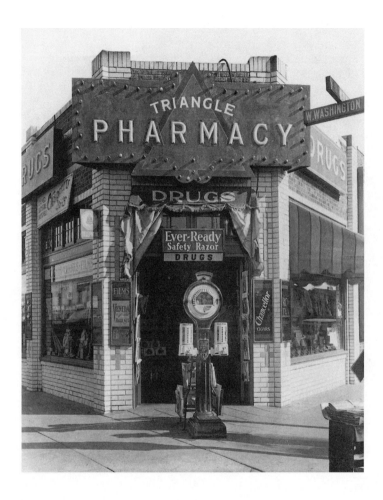

Los Angeles, 1920s. Drug stores have been a part of the commercial landscape for so long that we forget that they are also healthcare providers. *Courtesy of the University of Southern California, on behalf of the USC Library Department of Special Collections.*

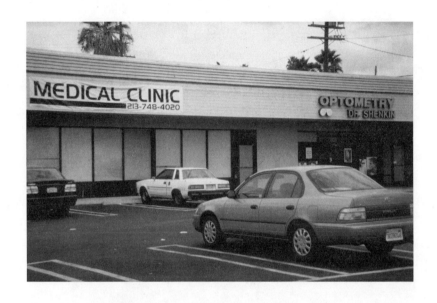

Los Angeles, 1990s. Accessible parking is one advantage of locating medical services in mini-malls. *Photograph by Beverlie Conant Sloane.*

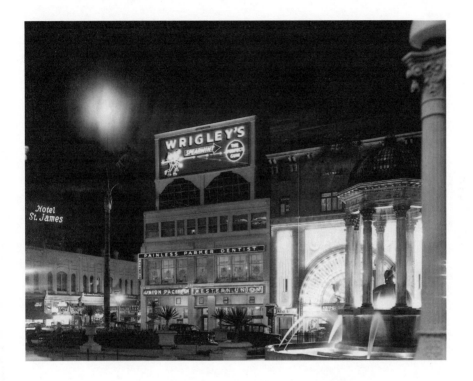

San Diego, California, 1935. Painless Parker was a rogue dentist who used advertising before it was socially and professionally acceptable for medical practitioners to do so. The brighly lit establishment next door houses the Turkish baths, apparently with doctor's and dentist's offices above them. *Courtesy of the San Diego Historical Society, Photograph Collection.*

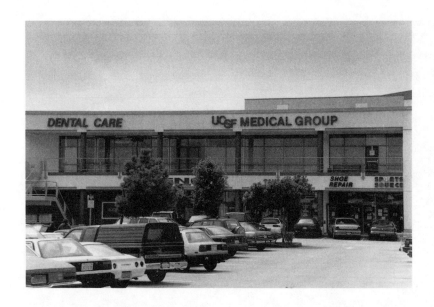

San Francisco, 1994. The Lakeshore Dental Care office and the University of California–San Francisco Medical Group satellite clinic are firmly part of the commercial scene in this busy urban shopping center. *Photograph by Beverlie Conant Sloane.*

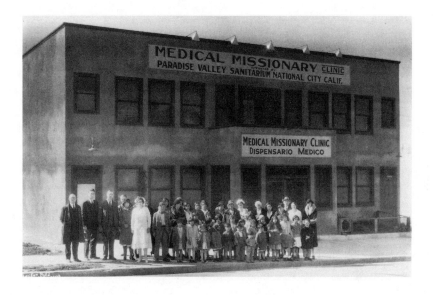

Outside San Diego, California, 1932. Early outpatient clinics served urban and rural poor families. The tone was often paternalistic. In this celebratory photograph of the opening of a medical missionary clinic in National City, the white male physicians stand next to but not among the patients they will be serving. *Courtesy of the San Diego Historical Society, Photograph Collection.*

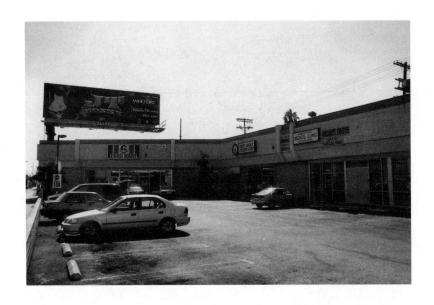

Los Angeles, 1990s. Many of the new mini-mall clinics continue the tradition that outpatient clinics serve primarily the poor. Among immigrants, medical insurance is an unusual employment benefit, so they depend on fee-for-service providers and are most likely to patronize those that locate in their neighborhoods. *Photograph by Beverlie Conant Sloane.*

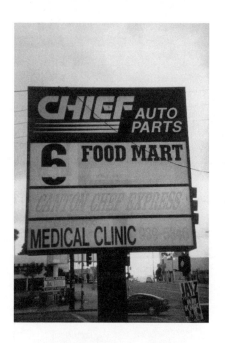

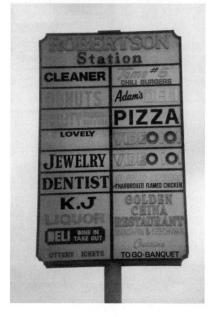

Los Angeles, 1980s. Mini-mall signs attest to the change in the medical landscape. The dentist and medical clinic fit snugly next to the auto parts store, doughnut shop, and liquor store. *Photographs by Beverlie Conant Sloane.*

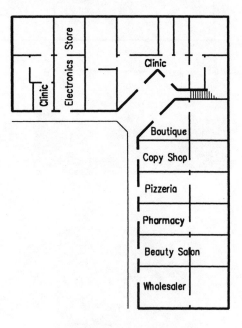

Los Angeles, 1980s. L-shaped plans like this one are
popular for strip malls and mini-malls, because they
provide for adequate parking and offer good visibility
to passing motorists.

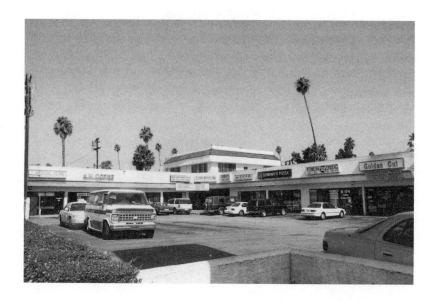

Los Angeles, 1980s. In multiethnic Los Angeles, the Van Ness Shopping Center houses a Korean pharmacy, a church-run clinic, a Latino botanica, and a satellite clinic from a primarily African American hospital. *Photograph by Beverlie Conant Sloane.*

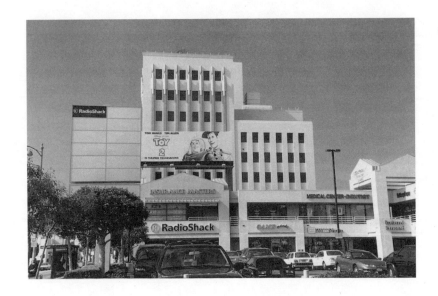

Los Angeles, 1980s. This mini-mall at Highland Avenue and Wilshire Boulevard has a more permanent look than smaller strip malls, but clinics like the one above the game store and photo shop come and go with frightening frequency. Hospitals may change and grow, but they rarely move. *Photograph by Beverlie Conant Sloane.*

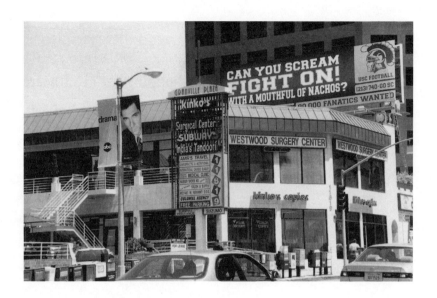

Los Angeles, 1988. Some forms of surgery are now more frequently occurring away from the hospital than in it. Will the public accept one-stop shopping for photocopies, a hamburger, a video game, and surgery? *Photograph by Beverlie Conant Sloane.*

THREE /   Shopping for Healthcare

The colors of two universities—the University of Southern California's cardinal and gold and the University of California at Los Angeles's blue and gold—can be found all around Los Angeles. These crosstown rivals compete on every level, from sports to alumni boasts. You can't go to a party without hearing some comment if you say you work for one or the other. Barbs even punctuate business meetings. The local television newscasts spend news time chronicling pep-rallying events the week prior to the annual USC-UCLA football game, and everything from commercial signs to license plate holders use the colors to proclaim allegiance and loyalty. Not surprisingly, in recent years, UCLA has employed this "name branding" to support its growing network of satellite primary care stand-alone clinics on Westside Los Angeles.

Strategically placed in the area's wealthier neighborhoods, these clinics are intended to serve both as accessible primary care centers and as feeders into the specialist practitioners at the massive UCLA Medical Center. The satellites typically move into offices previously used by a small clinic practice. Often UCLA has purchased the practice and incorporated it into their network. UCLA's expansion into the commercial marketplace has been controversial, their competitors arguing that the nonprofit university has an unfair advantage.[1] And, indeed, the clinics are hard to miss. Large blue-and-gold signs with "UCLA" prominently displayed announce them to passersby.

These satellite networks are partly a result of the outpatient revolution discussed in the previous chapter. While hospitals have been reinvented to maintain as much business at the medical center as possible, such satellite networks are quickly becoming standard practice nationwide. Hospital and medical center administrators are increasingly recognizing the necessity of reaching out to the public. In San Francisco, the University of California–San Francisco Medical Group has come down off "the Hill" and opened a satellite facility (with "UCSF" a prominent part of the display sign) in a shopping center. "In suburban Minneapolis, Group Health Inc., an HMO, has satellite clinics in four malls, including a 12,000-square-foot site in the giant Mall of America."[2] Even Dartmouth-Hitchcock Medical Center, which remains in rural New Hampshire, has opened a satellite clinic in a commercial building. Any large hospital is either considering satellite operations or has already implemented this strategy for drawing patients. Each new clinic represents the decentralized, commercialized medical landscape in which hospitals are searching for patients and patients are shopping for health.

Medicine in the Mini-Mall

These satellites are located in all sorts of places, from the first floor of a medical office building to a storefront shop next to a pizza place. Many are small stand-alone offices, dubbed "doc-in-a-box," situated in little commercial parks. A growing number are located in strip malls and mini-malls, places often reviled as the worst part of modern American cityscapes. In the American imagination, mini-malls are not proper sites for the serious concern of medicine. Often they are occupied by unstable businesses that frequently change owners and tenants, some looking as if at any moment they might close altogether. They do not seem fit places for confidential and personal affairs, where people can quietly seek advice about illness or fears of something worse. At their worst, these "highway strips" can be what New Urbanist advocate James Howard Kunstler calls "boulevards so horrible that every trace of human aspiration seems to have been expelled, except the impetus to sell."[3] Mini-malls and strip malls are the black sheep of the automotive city, necessary for its commerce but not important or serious enough for careful design or comprehensive planning. Certainly, most people would believe that they are not appropriate places for professionals to practice the sacred art of medicine.

Still, mini-malls and strip malls continue to multiply, as cities sprawl across the American countryside, and medicine spreads with them. The decentralization of healthcare facilities is especially evident in Los Angeles, the icon of the postwar automotive culture. Scholars have only cursorily examined the elements that are shaping this new landscape, the decentralization of commerce, and the spatial reorganization of American healthcare.[4] However, urban Americans, especially those in the South and West, will recognize the phenomenon. Indeed, they might view it as old hat. However, if they remember where they received their healthcare ten, even five years ago, they will realize how fast the landscape is changing.

The landscape is evolving because of changes in healthcare practices and competition, the maturation of the American drive-in culture, and the successful decentralization of such forerunners as dental and eye care and alternative medical care facilities. As the ways people navigate the city and the way they traverse the healthcare system change, healthcare managers are forced to reconsider their spatial relationships to their potential patients. Centralized medical facilities may offer tremendous economies of scale for the acute care of complex illnesses, but they are very often ill equipped to offer accessible, convenient care for routine health and preventive health procedures. Imagine instead a coordinated healthcare system, where well-baby visits, asthma shots, annual physicals, and other routine medical services are performed in a person's neighborhood, and only more serious illnesses are transferred to a community hospital or regional medical center. Paradoxically, even with all its potential problems, mini-mall medicine holds out that promise.

For some people, mini-mall medicine offers their only choice for care. Many new clinics have opened in poor, underserved neighborhoods. The clinics are often the only healthcare system for millions of uninsured or underinsured Americans who do not qualify for government programs but cannot afford private health insurance. The number of such Americans is staggering.[5] Their plight creates fertile ground for new private clinics, which locate in accessible and convenient places so that they can compete more successfully for patients. Unfortunately, these clinics are also especially vulnerable to the vagaries of healthcare economics. Many have closed, leaving patients adrift. Mini-mall medicine holds out the promise of accessibility, but potentially at the price of instability.

Changing Medical Practice

Physicians have moved to the mini-mall because the medical system is undergoing fundamental shifts that have made access, visibility, and expense increasingly important. First, competition in the healthcare system is fiercer than ever before. The healthcare market had long been constrained by regulations on admission into the profession, control of admitting privileges to hospitals, and a prohibition against advertising. Medicine was viewed, and its practitioners viewed themselves, as above, or at least outside, the marketplace. Employers' demands for discounted rates of care to hold down insurance costs and the constant discussions about federal healthcare subsidies for the elderly and poor have made the financial structures of healthcare much more visible to consumers and to the employers often paying for their insurance. The rise of the health maintenance organization (HMO) and other managed care organizations since the 1970s has fostered competition and encouraged conglomeration into healthcare systems, such as the hospital chains, like Health Care America, that have become so common. Many consumers have a choice every fall, when their employee benefits packages are reassessed, between competing plans and providers. To encourage subscriptions, plans must be visible, and systems need to compete for patients by ensuring that they offer low-cost and, hopefully, high-quality healthcare. Mini-mall medicine is part of a broader response to the new competition.

Second, competition has aggravated disparities in healthcare access and outcomes, and this also encourages mini-mall medicine. The privatization of hospitals and health systems shuts out those who cannot subscribe to those facilities. Managed care systems limit patients' choices, again diminishing options for everyone within the larger healthcare system. While managed care at least briefly leveled the exorbitant costs of healthcare, it has done little to address the crucial issue of access for poor working-class families and employees of small businesses burdened with the seemingly endless rounds of rises in insurance rates. Critics worry that managed care reduces access, lowers quality, and shifts cost containment to the physician, leaving patients in particularly vulnerable positions. One outcome is small "doc-in-a-box" clinics offering uninsured and underinsured families fee-for-care services.

The third critical change is the rise and remarkable expansion of ambulatory or outpatient services discussed in the last chapter. The rise in hospital outpatient visits alone has been dramatic, without counting the huge number of visits to group clinics and individual practices. In-patient medicine was the standard concern of twentieth-century medicine, but ambulatory care will replace it as healthcare's primary concern in the new century.

Because ambulatory medicine does not require that patients go to hospitals, it provides the incentive to decentralize care into less expensive quarters, such as those in small shopping centers or in stand-alone buildings along a commercial street.

A fourth shift has been the growing acceptance of complementary and alternative therapies. Americans have long used varieties of alternative medicine, ranging from chiropractors to acupuncturists. However, studies show that an increasing number of Americans view such treatments as legitimate and valid. A survey by the Center for Alternative Medicine Research and Education at Beth Israel Hospital and Harvard University estimates that while Americans already made roughly 387 million visits to practitioners of alternative therapies in 1990, the number skyrocketed to over 628 million in 1997.[6] Although alternative care providers continue to struggle for legitimacy within the medical profession, their growing popularity among the public reflects late-twentieth-century Americans' skepticism of conventional medicine. The two medical systems seem to coexist, or, as advocates are hoping, to complement, each other, with indications that many Americans use them each interchangeably, depending on their illness.

The expansion of alternative medicine may also be tied to the rise of the competitive medical marketplace, which has left many Americans with inadequate healthcare insurance and continually frustrated with the conventional healthcare system. In the past twenty years, Americans have become much more willing to accept the legitimacy of such practitioners, and so have insurance companies, conventional practitioners, and the rest of the mainstream healthcare system. The National Institutes of Health have an institute focusing on alternative, or complementary, care. Harvard Medical School and other prominent medical schools have active research programs looking at the efficacy of alternative treatments. The success of alternative care further complicates the medical marketplace, especially spatially, since alternative practitioners have long been located in more-commercial sites. Ironically, conventional practitioners may have to move to the commercial districts of their cities to be as visible as are alternative therapists.

The shifts in competitiveness, place of care, and types of care all reinforce the spread of mini-mall medicine. The competitive market for health consumers encourages the relocation of primary care and some specialty care to facilities more convenient to potential patients. The places where consumers spend their daily lives are along the boulevards and in the neighborhood shopping centers.

From Home to Office

The new commercial landscape represents quite a change from the older city. While changes in medical practice and financing provide a rationale for the relocation of medicine, the sites it now occupies reflect the impact of the automobile on the built landscape. In one of his last papers, landscape scholar John Brinckerhoff Jackson stated in 1990 that the "car has taken over . . . taking the family to the day care center, the laundromat, the supermarket, the drive-in restaurant, the emergency room at the hospital." Jackson argued that "what makes most American cities interesting . . . is that . . . they are not pedestrian cities; they are not to be explored on foot."[7] The automobile extends the city, opening its horizons even as it sprawls over the land, stretching "for miles and miles" over the great boulevards, such as those in Los Angeles.

The regional shopping mall is the most prominent symbol of the decentralization of retail shopping. The downtown is no longer the dominant commercial center, only one of many retail nodes spread throughout the metropolitan area. These nodes, though, are only the prime retail attractions. Just as dozens of smaller specialty stores used to surround downtown department stores, today's retail and cultural centers are part of a linked web of services. This web is often taken for granted. To grab a bag of chips, Americans head for the convenience store connected to the gas station. Needing our toaster fixed or a new towel rack, Americans drive over to a small neighborhood shop that stands alongside several others in a small shopping district on a major street near their neighborhood. Looking for basic ingredients, they drive a bit further to a grocery store in a larger shopping center, usually fronted by a large parking lot. On special occasions, when they want to be entertained, or to choose from a larger set of shopping choices, they travel to the shopping mall or to downtown.

Of course, this hierarchy is only an idealized picture. In the early days of the twentieth century, downtown was truly dominant, and if you wanted a specialty item you had to go there. But, now people shop for daily needs, such as groceries, in the shopping mall, and go to local commercial streets

140

for items not available in the mall. Or they don't go out at all; they have their groceries delivered, get their clothes from a catalogue, buy books off the Internet, and purchase specialty items from home shopping shows on television. Still, most people don't shop at home. The street, whether paved by the city or invented by retailers, is the place to find goods and services. Street or mall, the hierarchy of stores is no longer clearly defined.

Medical practice has always had a place within the commercial network. Dentists could be found along commercial streets, as well as pharmacists, optometrists, chiropractors, and herbalists. Outpatient clinics for the poor were located in or near commercial districts. But all of these commercial sites were marginal to the main focus of the medical profession, which maintained its distance from the commercial world. Self-imposed regulations severely constrained the use of advertising and carefully screened practitioners through licensing, privileges, and other procedures. When medical practice did appear along the commercial streets, it did so in the dignified and differentiated space of the medical office building.

Although some physicians still maintain home offices, American physicians largely practiced from their homes prior to the twentieth century. The increasing sophistication of medical technology, medicine's avowal of science, and the hospital's primacy encouraged them to move to other quarters. They did not move into the hospital, as many might assume today. Physicians were more likely to move into offices in small professional buildings near hospitals or in the many speculative office buildings sprouting up in America's downtowns. The introduction of steel framing, the elevator, and other building innovations set the stage for a boom in office construction. Offices were concentrated in downtown areas, creating street canyons between increasingly higher office mountains. For instance, Los Angeles has the Broadway Central Building, a ten-story steel and concrete structure opened in 1908. Among its original tenants were ten physicians, four dentists, and one oral surgeon, along with a Christian Science practitioner, an osteopathic physician, and the offices of the California Medical and Electric Institute and the American Hospital Association, which was an early, local health insurance operation.[8] Retailers, businesses, and wholesalers filled the other offices in this $300,000 speculative downtown structure.

Accompanying the description of the Broadway Central Building in the *American Globe*, a local progressive monthly, was an article describing one building tenant's practice in "oral surgery." Dr. C. Deichmiller convinced the reporter that if "people knew [of] the possibilities" of his "comparatively new" but "useful" specialty, few would, in the words of the reporter, "apply in these cases to general practitioners of dentistry." Specialization was transforming medicine. It propelled the development of new medical spaces, since these physicians desired to separate themselves from general practitioners and often referred patients to each other. Of course, referrals would come only through appropriate means. As Dr. Deichmiller told the reporter, he was "in the strict ethical class of practitioners who frown at the mere mention of advertising or publicity." He stood outside the crass commercial world even as he inhabited offices on a busy downtown street. This oral surgeon, like so many other physicians, maintained that his professionalism mandated his superiority over that world.

The trend towards specialization that had begun in the late nineteenth century pervaded American medicine in the post–World War II era, encouraging the development of further medical office facilities. In 1949, 75 percent of physicians were general practitioners or specialists in internal medicine and pediatrics, specialties largely involved in primary care. By 1983, only 39 percent of physicians were in those three categories. At the same time, the number of physicians was increasing, tripling between 1950 and 1987.[9] Specialization encouraged the creation of group practices, often tied to specific hospitals. As David McBride argues, starting in the 1930s, "the tendency by the majority of private GP's (general practitioners) to perpetuate their own individually housed practices waned, and the delivery of medical care in Philadelphia and other cities became progressively centralized around the hospitals." As healthcare expert Milton I. Roemer asserted, in this new age of specialization, these office buildings were part of a "rationalization of ambulatory medical care by way of group practice clinics" that became much more familiar to Americans after World War II.[10]

Medical office buildings were opened to serve families and individuals who could no longer expect a doctor to make a house call and who wanted the best possible care that the expanding medical system could offer. The same buildings might hold eye care, dental care, physical or occupational therapy, and other related medical services, as well as physicians' offices. Often called the Medical Arts Building, these structures proliferated throughout the United States. Americans came to expect that a visit to the doctor would happen as typically in an office building as anywhere else.

In Los Angeles, dozens of such buildings were constructed throughout the twentieth century. Some, such as the Wilshire Metropolitan Medical Center (now the Samaritan Medical Towers), were located on the great commercial boulevards. According to a contemporary advertisement, the office building, which opened in 1964 on perhaps the nation's most famous mid-twentieth century boulevard, was sited "just west of the Harbor Freeway and easy to get to from any point in the Southland." It was convenient to "ALL major Los Angeles hospitals," with suites "tailored to meet the individual doctor's specialized needs."[11] The sleek concrete and glass fifteen-story building gave no indication that it was dedicated to the medical arts. Instead, its dark glass doorway offered only an opaque window to the passing cars. Along the long corridors of offices within the building, small signs announced the available medical services. Discreet practices sheltered from the commercial world outside.

As the city sprawled outward, medical practice followed, along with other social institutions, such as churches and fraternal groups. In the suburbanized metropolis, new sites were available for medical entrepreneurship. Trying to reach a wider audience of consumers, healthcare institutions opened facilities in places they would have ignored a decade before. Suburban sites were now desirable, and convenience took on increased importance. Fewer and fewer hospitals were being constructed downtown. Instead, the federal Hill-Burton legislation funded hundreds of suburban hospitals nationwide, contributing to a new, suburban infrastructure. The majority of new hospitals were being built in the expanding suburbs, as were the airports, office building centers, industrial sites, and homes. Examples in Southern California included Daniel Freeman Hospital in Marina Del Rey, St. Joseph's Hospital in Orange, and St. Jude's Hospital in Fullerton.

Many doctor's offices congregated around these hospitals. An example of this type of agglomeration occurred in one of Boston's western suburbs, Needham, around Deaconness Grover Hospital. Two stand-alone medical office buildings appeared near the hospital, which is one-quarter mile from the suburb's commercial center. In addition, a primary care wellness center is situated behind and above retail stores. A specialty ambulatory clinic is located in a larger building that also houses a video store, an assisted living residence, a skilled nursing facility, and a community dental office side-by-side with a real estate firm. This suburban grouping is a microcosm of such congregations around hospitals in nearly every American city, with much larger aggregations around renowned medical districts like Boston's Longwood, with its numerous hospitals and ancillary offices.

Southern California physicians who had taken offices in the prestigious downtown buildings found they were competing with doctors in buildings more conveniently located to the families who used them. The Los Altos Medical Building (now Buildings), located in Los Angeles County just south of the famed 1950s suburb of Lakewood, is an example of the suburbanizing of medicine.[12] The original architects, Kite and Overpeck, customized its suites, which boasted air conditioning, easy access to the San Diego Freeway, Class-A construction, and on-site radiology and pathology laboratories. The two-story, multisection structure sported canopied walkways between the building sections. Its horizontal design mirrored the nearby suburban residential neighborhoods, while its glass and concrete construction reflected the materials of business and industry. Inside such buildings, around the nation, the medical practice was invisible to the outside, undefined and unseen from the road. The professional medical office building had joined the commercial scene, but strictly on its own terms.

Emergence of the Mini-Mall

Careful isolation of medical services in a separate building from retail commodities is quickly fading.[13] As the boundaries between professional and retail services have blurred, medicine can be found anywhere. A dentist may locate in an upper floor of a professional building or the corner of a shopping center. A medical clinic may be situated next to the photocopy shop or in a stand-alone building on the edge of a fashionable residential area. An acupuncturist may have an office upstairs from a chiropractor in a corner mini-mall or in a small, adapted residential structure on a busy commercial street. A "surgicenter" may open opposite a fast-food restaurant or nestle next to the medical center. In the current commercial city, healthcare providers may share space with virtually any retail business.

They are becoming especially evident along the broad, endless urban boulevards that have in many cities become home to the strip mall or its compact counterpart, the mini-mall. With a rising torrent of commerce and automobiles along the commercial street, both consumers and retailers have been caught in the current. In the words of John Brinckerhoff Jackson, modern-day "mobile consumers" "think nothing of traveling to a supermarket that has better parking than one located two miles nearer." The flexibility and convenience of the car alter space and place. Retailers "must learn to attract . . . business in a way they never had to do when customers were confined to a certain familiar area."[14] For a business simply to have a good name, even a reasonable location, is no longer enough; the marketplace has become too competitive.

The battle for retail recognition in the increasingly fast urban world has shaped many commercial trends during the twentieth century. Fighting for space, attention, and customers, retailers have strung themselves out over miles of streets, looking to be more accessible, more attractive, more easily noticed, and more profitable. Parking became a major issue as early as the 1920s, and it has only increased in importance since.[15] The car created convenience but diminished recognizability. Imagine someone trying to pick out an address or a sign while walking at 3 miles per hour compared to driving at 30, 40, or 50 miles per hour. The visual signals have to be very bold and eye-catching.

Architects and planners Venturi, Scott Brown, and Izenour dissected this landscape in their brilliant analysis of Las Vegas. Although many critics have argued that "the commercial strip is chaos," they found a particular order. Critical to that order is the contrast between street and building. The civic zone of the street represents a "shared order" that everyone recognizes. Streets provide entrances and exits in a very orderly fashion. The private, individualized zone of the building allows for variety and change. Service stations to casinos, marriage chapels to luxury hotels, the buildings create a different kind of order, one derived from their particular nexus and their constant reference to the automobile and its street. Together the buildings and signs embrace "continuity *and* discontinuity, going *and* stopping, clarity *and* ambiguity, cooperation *and* competition, the community *and* rugged individualism."[16] The commercial strip is visually ordinary, even ugly; but it is also representative of American culture and society, a merger of the civic and individual, the communal and personal.

The development of the mini-mall is symbolic of this bolder, auto-centered commercial landscape. As historian Richard Longstreth persuasively argues in his studies of Los Angeles's commercial architecture, the development of the small neighborhood shopping center spans the automotive age.[17] The building type has evolved through the decades, changing parking configurations, altering tenant mixes and adapting to the latest architectural fashions. Throughout, the neighborhood center has served a local market with convenience goods. Today, instead of a small grocery store and shoe emporium, one often finds a video store and a restaurant, but the purpose of the commerce has changed very little.

Convenience was the foundation for the proliferation of a new type of small shopping center, variously called "corner malls" because they were often located on busy intersections, "podmalls" for their pod-like look and construction techniques, and "mini-malls" since they carried forward on a smaller scale the lessons learned in the larger shopping malls. In Los Angeles, the mini-mall began to appear in the 1970s.[18] La Mancha Development Corporation, the city's foremost early mini-mall builder, constructed its first mini-mall in 1972 in Panorama City in the San Fernando Valley on the site of a recently closed gas station. Perhaps as many as 3,000 gas stations were forced to close in Los Angeles in the 1970s and 1980s due to the OPEC oil embargo and the end of oil company subsidies. Since many of them were located on corner lots at busy intersections, developers experimented with replacing them with corner convenience centers.

The centers were "a cluster of [retail] specialists that neighbors could visit without spending hours at a large mall or driving from one street to another."[19] Being on the corner was critical. Los Angeles's planning officials argued that the mini-malls were so successful because, while the "old pattern of commercial development was along the highways," now "its at intersections inside the city." At intersections, working mothers could stop on the way home to pick up that last item for dinner, or teens driving home from school could stop to pick up a soda and snacks. Given the mobile, fragmented social lives of many Angelinos, convenience had become a major sales advantage. The large shopping malls were great as destinations but a parking nightmare for a quick purchase. The great commercial streets suffered from the same parking problem. They were especially hurt by transportation "improvements" that forbade parking during peak commuter hours. The quart of milk might cost an extra dime or more at a mini-mall, but the perceived savings in time and inconvenience were well worth it. As a result, by the mid-1980s, officials reported that as many as 2,000 mini-malls had been constructed throughout Los Angeles, reshaping the commercial environment. The number had increased to roughly 3,000 just five years later. A booming economy and the changing social habits of American families fueled the mini-mall boom.

Immigration also played a critical role in maintaining the expansion of mini-malls throughout the city. During the 1990s, Los Angeles and California became national exemplars of the politics and economics of immigration. Proposition 187, the economic border wars along the Rio Grande, and the growing visibility of Latinos in state and local politics are all examples of this phenomenon. The numbers of immigrants to the city are staggering. The region grew from roughly 10 million to 14.5 million between 1970 and 1990. Much of this population increase was fueled by international immigration, particularly from Mexico and Central America and Southeast Asia. By 2000, the city of Los Angeles had become a majority Latino city.

The new immigrants are known for working extremely hard to meet the needs of their families. For example, even confronted with widespread ethnic-based discrimination, virtually all surveys show that almost every able-bodied Latino man works, even if his earnings are so small he must work two or three jobs to support a family. Asian families combine earnings and efforts to purchase or start many small businesses. Both groups of immigrants were eager applicants for spaces in the aggressively marketed mini-malls. They turned their hands to new jobs, and, as did earlier waves of immigrants, they brought skills and knowledge from their places of origin. "[Immigrants] want what they had in the old country," observed Sam Bachner, a leading mini-mall developer, asking, "How does a little Jewish man be a herbologist? Little Jewish men don't know from herbs. . . . These Orientals, they know from herbs."[20] Soon, mini-mall restaurants sprouted around the city, as did a variety of specialty shops, and health-related businesses.

Pharmacies

Pharmacists, alternative practitioners, optometrists, podiatrists, and community dentists have long situated themselves close to customers and among retailers, and they were the first to move into mini-malls.[21] These practitioners need to be conveniently located near consumers, especially in a highly competitive market, and they have less need for the technology and other benefits of proximity to a hospital. They have also had fewer professional barriers between them and the public. Starting out on commercial streets, they have found homes among the dry cleaners and the restaurants in the mini-malls, strip malls, shopping centers, and even regional shopping malls. They have constantly balanced the need for more visible commercial sites and new market realities with professional standards and ethics.

Pharmacies or drug stores are so much a part of the commercial healthcare landscape that Americans take for granted that they can be found there. However, they are a wonderful example of pioneering inclusion in the commercial healthcare landscape, and a possible model for future activities. Drugs have long been a crucial element in medicine. While early physicians almost always mixed their own nostrums, an allied profession gradually emerged to supplement their concoctions and to offer standardized potions. Although many pharmacies were owned and operated by physicians, other commercial or community drug stores provided medicines directly to the consumer. In that role, they became physically separated from doctors' offices, bringing them into the commercial landscape.

American pharmacies (or drug stores, the less professional, more popular term) have a legacy that stretches back to the colonial period. Most early drug stores were part of a general store or of a physician's practice. By the antebellum period, hundreds of apothecaries (a colonial term for a pharmacy) had been established throughout the United States. Most were in cities, and they often served as manufacturers for rural medical practices. In California in 1852, a report for the nascent American Pharmaceutical Association stated that "two-thirds of all the drug stores . . . are kept by physicians." However, the expertise afforded by physician ownership was balanced by professional instability. For example, a pharmacy in Baltimore was opened originally in 1849, by a recently graduated physician who was also a house carpenter. A few years later, he left the medical profession and sold the drug store to another doctor, who took on an apprentice. Shortly thereafter, the new owner left to become a lawyer, leaving the young apprentice, with barely two years of experience, as the sole owner of the drug store.[22]

In the nation's frontier cities, pharmacies often were forced to exchange drugs for barter. As early as the mid-nineteenth century, these exchanges led to the combination drug store, general store, and wholesale establishment that became representative of drug stores in the twentieth century. In this more retail atmosphere, not surprisingly, price competition and advertising became common. "Cut-rate" drug stores were established in the nation's growing cities, leading to the entry of entrepreneurs into the drug store business. Legislative lobbying by independent drug store associations limited the full extent of the drug market for much of the twentieth century, but could not stop the development of a broad retail competition. Originally, druggists themselves compounded most of the pharmaceutical products they sold. By the 1970s, manufacturers made virtually all drugs, with drug stores serving as dispensing retail establishments. Supermarkets and other retail establishments realized the potential for selling a limited number of popular drugs in the 1950s, which created further competition to independent pharmacies. And, drug store chains, pioneered by Louis K. Liggett and Charles R. Walgreen in the early years of the twentieth century, proved even greater competition. Walgreen, for instance, opened his first pharmacy in 1901. He expanded to 9 stores in 1916, 462 in 1961, and 580 (plus almost 2000 franchised outlets) in 1973.

The modern discount drug stores are ubiquitous in the commercial healthcare landscape. They can be found in stand-alone stores on the great commercial strips as well as in regional shopping malls, pod malls, mini-malls, strip malls, and neighborhood commercial districts. In addition, pharmacies are now an expected unit of large grocery stores. In the 1990s, they often took up ever-larger space, as prescription drug sales were combined with herbal products and an assortment of associated healthcare products to develop health centers. Many strip malls have chain drug stores, while larger shopping centers are more likely to have the new super or mega drug stores.

In some poor Latino communities, drug stores, known typically as *botanicas*, serve a variety of purposes. They offer not only prescription drugs but also herbal medicines and a range of healthcare advice. They are likely not to be franchises of the large drug store chains. They are typically small stores, often in strip or mini-malls, like the *botanica* in the Van Ness Plaza on Pico Boulevard. This *botanica* shares space with two clinics and a Korean pharmacy, as well as a hair salon and pizza place. Some Latino drug stores have been accused of serving as informal healthcare facilities, where poor people go for inexpensive medical care. Pharmacists offer medical advice and give shots, leading to problems that will be discussed in a later section of this chapter.

Alternative Medicine

Through most of American history, medicine, "conventional or allopathic medicine," coexisted with many alternative theories of care.[23] Hydrotherapy, homeopathy, and other alternative therapeutic systems were widely practiced in the years before the Civil War. Chinese herbalists have been dispensing solutions since they arrived on the West Coast in the middle decades of the nineteenth century. With the advent of medical licensing legislation in the late nineteenth century and the tightening of professional regulations in the early twentieth century, alternative therapies were greatly constrained. They could continue to operate but under increasing scrutiny and restrictions. Practitioners of alternative medicine were rarely invited inside the medical office buildings or allowed to admit patients into hospitals. Instead, they thrived in ethnic commercial areas, such as the local Chinatown and Little Tokyo, or operated out of private residences and in small out-of-the-way commercial storefront shops.

A generation ago, few Americans could describe acupuncture or would venture into an herbal medicine store. The most acceptable alternative therapy, chiropractic, was well known but still quite controversial. Now, this huge alternative care system is spreading and becoming more visible and more accepted. Almost 34 percent of American adults made a visit to an alternative medicine practitioner in 1990, while just over 42 percent did so in 1997. Americans paid out-of-pocket expenses of over $12 billion to alternative medicine practitioners, $5.1 billion for herbal therapies, $3.3 billion for megavitamins, $1.7 billion on alternative therapy-specific books, classes, and equipment, for an estimated total of $27 billion. In comparison, Americans paid an estimated $9 billion for hospitalizations and $29.3 billion in out-of-pocket expenses to conventional physicians.[24]

The local and national figures suggest that the much-vaunted alternative medicine revolution is actually over, Americans having accepted a wide range of therapies that they perceive as beneficial to them. They look to alternative practitioners when conventional medicine fails them, either by not providing an effective treatment or by treating them dispassionately. As one new age practitioner stated, "Many alternative medical treatments are 'a lot like the way medicine used to be.'"[25] People do not turn to alternative therapies for all the illnesses for which they might consult a conventional doctor. Still, the range is impressive, from obesity and a variety of weight-related conditions to muscular injuries often presumed to require surgery. For instance, of those reporting that they had back problems, 48 percent had used some alternative therapy during the previous year to relieve it and 30 percent had gone to see an alternative therapy practitioner during the same period. Backaches may seem an obvious example, especially with the increased reliance on chiropractors, but 12 percent had used a therapy to combat high blood pressure, 13 percent to prevent insomnia, 41 percent to fight depression, and 27 percent to treat arthritis. For many Americans, alternative medicine practitioners serve as an important supplement to conventional medicine. As alternative methods are increasingly accepted by the medical and insurance establishments, they are being referred to as "complementary" medicine.

Alternative therapies are not uniformly distributed around the United States. Healthcare researcher Shri Mishra reports that not only do Californians use alternative medicine services at a rate much higher than the national estimates, but that those services are unevenly located throughout Southern California. Comparing a national and state poll of use, Mishra found that Californians used chiropractic, homeopathic, and acupuncture services roughly twice as often as national estimates. Alternative medicine practitioners cluster near these potential patients. Mishra mapped the location of acupuncturists and chiropractors in Los Angeles County. He found acupuncturists in three large areas that have very different ethnic compositions. One is largely white, the second Latino, and the last Asian. Chiropractic offices are more evenly distributed throughout the city and county, but they tend to be in areas that are predominantly white.[26]

Alternative medicine practitioners see patients in every conceivable type of medical facility. Near the Los Angeles International Airport, in the area of Westchester, is a new three-building shopping center anchored by a large grocery store. Various retail outlets—video, pet care, café, and other restaurants—are in a two-story stucco building that blocks the grocery store from the street. On the second floor, above the pet care store, is a chiropractic clinic. Across town one finds a very different example. In a vaguely Mediterranean-style commercial building are two stores facing one the area's busiest streets, in the heart of an immigrant community. In one storefront is a Salvadoran and Mexican restaurant; in the other an acupuncturist advertising in English and Korean. These two settings are among dozens of mini-malls, commercial storefronts, and even regional shopping malls with alternative medicine practitioners.

Limited Medical Practitioners

The third group that pioneered in the retail marketplace are sometimes called "limited medical practitioners," because they concentrate on one portion of the body. Podiatrists work solely on feet, dentists on teeth and gums, and optometrists on eyes. They are recognized by their fellow physicians as experts in their areas of expertise but are often not given full professional status, since they have specialized training programs. In each case, other practitioners, such as orthopedic surgeons and opthamologists, also have interest in the area of expertise and greater professional status. In the institutional structure of twentieth-century medicine, the limited medical practitioners have established themselves, but often at the margins of medical practice. For instance, they might be included in a medical office building, although usually on the first floor with the retail services rather than on the upper, clinical floors. In recent years, though, as the medical marketplace has opened up and regulations have been eased, these practitioners have become much more visible in the medical landscape.

Dental offices are, after pharmacies, perhaps the most common medical service in the commercial landscape. Although dentists have been able to retain a highly prestigious professional standing, and their services are covered by optional health insurance, they have not been enmeshed in the hospital web. Instead, dental offices have long been community-based. Los Angeles dentists could be found in home-based offices and office buildings early in the twentieth century. However, dental associations were formed to maintain professional standards and ethics that included limiting advertising and mandating the independence of practitioners.

Recently, Arden G. Christen and Peter M. Pronych authored a fascinating biography of Painless Parker, a dentist who rebelled against these standards.[27] Parker was active on both coasts, eventually creating a dental empire based in San Francisco and Los Angeles in the 1910s. Parker advertised heavily, including very gaudy promotional circus acts that offended and appalled his contemporaries. Painless Parker dental offices were opened in five states, employing dozens of dentists. His slogan, "All Operations Performed Absolutely Without Pain," became known to a generation of West Coast residents. Dental associations largely scorned his activities as demeaning to the profession. However extreme his antics became—and his association with high-wire acts and magic potions was pretty wild—he and other pioneers blazed the trail for the modernization of business practices. When, in the 1970s, the Federal Trade Commission (FTC) prohibited professional associations' bans on advertising by their members, Parker's empire was long gone, but advertising became accepted practice.

Dentists have not yet faced the franchising and consolidation that has occurred in so many other health service sectors. Numerous dentists are still independent operators, with their offices in their homes. Others have moved into a medical office or a mixed commercial building. In Los Angeles's Koreatown, the California Medical Group's two-story reinforced concrete building houses health services ranging from internal medicine and obstetrics to acupuncture and dentistry. As anyone driving around any town or city can attest, dentists are occupying more commercially advantageous spaces, including mini-malls. A short drive north of the University of Southern California, West Coast Dental is located in a shopping center in a structure separated from the main building, which holds a large grocery store. West Cost Dental's banner, "Free Braces Exam," competes for attention with the neighboring video store's movie posters. A few miles away, in the elongated Venice Boulevard strip mall named Robertson Station, whose one-story brick façade covers almost an entire city block, a community dental practice is surrounded by such commercial businesses as jewelry, video, liquor, and manicure stores, as well as restaurants and offices. In the jumbled buildings of Baldwin Hills Center, located on one of the city's busiest commuter streets, La Brea Boulevard, a dental center sits on the upper floor of a very plain concrete building fronted by a long parking lot.

The discreet medical signage of the past, in which doctors' names were welded in small letters on brass plaques affixed to the sides of buildings, or institutions' names were etched into the glass doors of their offices, is giving way to more prominent advertising, new reach-out efforts, and even direct mail and telephone marketing. As late as the 1970s, patients could not shop for eyeglasses in some states, because they were legally prohibited from obtaining a copy of their prescription. Advertising among optometrists was frowned upon, if not, as in some states, illegal. And, optometrists were restricted from working for an optician or a chain of eyewear stores, for fear that they would lose their professional independence. Pioneers were castigated, then sued for trying to franchise and aggressively advertise their services.

In the new competitive healthcare market, under the revised FTC rules, advertising is an accepted part of professional trade, further blurring the commercial-professional boundary line. Eyecare entrepreneurs gradually forced states to remove restrictions to franchising, advertising, and one-stop shopping. Dr. Stanley Pearle "opened his first chain of stores in Georgia because his home state of Texas still prohibited corporate ownership of multiple sites by an optometrist." Within a few years, he and others had revolutionized the way Americans purchase glasses and contacts. Now eyecare stores are in all types of commercial spaces. They can be found in professional office buildings, mini-malls, shopping centers, and regional shopping malls. The various franchises, in addition to regional chains and individual providers, have become so much a part of the retail landscape, that they are no longer seen as a violation of professional ethics and practice.[28]

Still, they were pioneers. Eyecare shops that combine medical and retail services, offering both eye examinations and retail lenses and frames, are a model for the changing provision of primary and specialty medical services. Consumers have a wide range of choices, prices are comparable to other consumer goods, and lenses are now available within an hour of the exam. Eyecare practitioners have proven, by their example, that medical services can be provided efficiently and accessibly outside the hospital and medical office building. Obviously, some medical procedures are more adaptable to this model than others, and quality assurance is a serious concern. Still, the shift in eyecare delivery is suggestive of the potential development of mini-mall medicine.

Medical Clinicians in the Mini-Mall

While the pioneers have been located in commercial districts or shopping centers for some time, newcomers to the mini-mall and strip mall—primary care clinics, even specialty clinics—are beginning to open in such places in many American cities. In recent visits to the suburbs of Boston, Massachusetts, Bradenton, Florida, and Albany, New York, we found clinics in highly visible strip malls and set-back commercial buildings. In general, the clinics' locations reflect the inequities that continue to pervade the modern American healthcare system, as well as the expansion of the ambulatory healthcare system and the large hospitals' recognition of the need for satellite feeder systems. The decentralization of health services is occurring everywhere in urban and suburban America.

The emerging social geography of medicine is illustrated by two clinics not far from each other in Latham, New York, north of Albany. The first clinic is housed in a grand Federal-style mansion that reflects the heritage of the area and ties the practitioner to that history. The clinic is carefully designed to obscure its commercial nature; its parking area is carefully screened from passing cars, and its only sign is a short, barely visible stand-alone panel. Not more than one-half mile away, the Medical Surgical Center is located in Newton Plaza, one of several large strip malls clustered along Route 9. This classic example of a "doc-in-a-box" has a blue-lettered sign that competes with the neighboring ones for a liquor store and banking services. The center offers a wide range of ambulatory and pediatric services, including help for minor emergencies, routine physical exams, immunizations, and laboratory work. The office sign emphasizes its availability: "No Appointment Necessary!!!" So, a visitor could get a blood pressure check then visit the bagel shop, gift store, art gallery, and bookstore before picking up any necessary medicine at the pharmacy. The half-mile between these two clinics covers a long distance in the changing healthcare landscape.

The two clinics potentially represent the continuation of inequities as well as the changing location of medicine in the new healthcare landscape. The grand mansion may well serve commercially insured patients from the upper and middle class in the rapidly growing suburbs north of New York's capital city. The strip mall surgical center may well provide fee-for-service treatments for uninsured or underinsured rural and suburban working-class New Yorkers. Readers need little reminder that the American healthcare system continues to be economically and racially and ethnically inequitable. Historians, including Vanessa Gamble and David McBride, have documented the long struggle of African Americans to receive hospital and healthcare services, not only in the South, but throughout the United States. McBride reported that in 1956, while the ratio of residents to physicians in Los Angeles's white community was one to 355; in the black community it was one to 2,104. That was much better than in New Orleans or Atlanta, but still a frightening comment on America's racial inequities.[29] Today, the situation remains serious. Studies question why African Americans and other residents in poor urban neighborhoods, as well as poor whites in rural counties, receive different levels of certain types of care and continue to suffer from differences in quantity and quality of available medical services.

Not surprisingly, then, many mini-mall clinics are in poorer neighborhoods. In Southern California, this relocation is the result of the shuttering of public clinics, the restriction of some emergency rooms to insured customers, and the opportunity for private providers to receive governmental payments. Los Angeles County has one of the highest rates of uninsured residents in the nation. In 1997/98, experts estimated that fewer than 60 percent of workers there were covered by employer-based health insurance. Even when offered the insurance, many low-paid workers decline, because the employee's share is too expensive. As Juan T. Martinez told his employer when he was offered a policy that would cost him $350 a month, "What! You want my check for one week?"[30] A quarter of his pay would have been going toward health insurance. Among the city's working immigrant populations, especially the Southeast Asians and the Latinos, the rate of uninsured adults seems to be rising. Too many new jobs are part-time, seasonal, or too low paying to offer the "luxury" of health insurance. So, families look for private providers who offer inexpensive rates.

These families often use freestanding clinics that offer inexpensive medical services. Some such clinics are satellites of hospitals or group practices. One medical administrator told us about overseeing the development of nine satellite clinics in Chicago in the 1980s. They opened in a variety of locations, ranging from a renovated bank building to a strip mall with free front parking. Another clinic was installed in a commercial storefront across from a shopping mall, since the administrator viewed the mall as a magnet that would draw people to the entire commercial area.[31] By the mid-1990s, many satellite clinics were opening around the nation.

Other clinics are stand-alone practices nicknamed "doc-in-a-boxes." These small clinics have become pervasive in poorer neighborhoods of Los

Angeles. Driving down major commercial streets one may find a half-dozen such medical clinics. Some, such as the obstetric and pediatric clinics in a two-story concrete office building on Vermont Avenue near Koreatown, are in freestanding structures along commercial streets. Others, like the small medical office in a small one-story strip mall situated perpendicular to Figueroa Avenue a few blocks west of a major freeway, are nuzzled into commercial markets. Access, reasonable rents, and convenience seem to propel their choice of location.

Most clinics are isolated storefronts amid many other businesses. In a few places the medical services are agglomerating. The Van Ness Plaza shopping center is located in a low-income Latino neighborhood near the very busy transportation corridor of Vermont Avenue. It is a one-story, L-shaped center with a front parking lot. Its nondescript stucco façade is ornamented with a single wide blue stripe. A Drew University health clinic sits a few doors down from the St. Basil's health clinic, a private nonprofit provider. A third facility, Clinica Medica Familiar, is next to Yogi's Botanica and a pharmacy. The sign for the pharmacy is in English and Korean, suggesting the multiethnic clientele the center serves. Private and public, conventional and alternative are all tucked in neatly next to Domino's Pizza and the photocopying place.

These clinics serve many people who have been left out of the commercial American health insurance system. Other clinics clearly seek employed, insured patients in wealthier areas of the city. Many of these facilities are the freestanding structures along commercial avenues exemplified by the UCLA clinics discussed in the chapter opening. Mini-mall clinics, though, are growing in number. For example, at the corner of Highland Avenue and Wilshire Boulevard is a mini-mall that is representative of the newer architectural styles, with a two-story layout in a Mediterranean style with a pseudo-postmodern cupola. The center is located just east of a successful commercial street at the heart of a diverse neighborhood flanked by a wealthy residential area to the east and Museum Row to the west. The center has an interesting mix of stores that serve local residents and nearby businesses on Wilshire and La Brea. The classic mini-mall categories are all covered: fast food at Fatburgers and Subway, Kinko's photocopy services, the beauty salon and the dry cleaners, and semiprofessional services at the insurance agent. Set amidst them are the medical services: a dentist, a small medical clinic, a massage therapist, a chiropractor, and an acupuncturist.

Similarly, in 1994 the University of California at San Francisco Medical Group opened a large satellite clinic in a U-shaped shopping center in the city's Sunset District. The gleaming white panels contrast with the large bright blue UCSF letters on the second-story façade. Those large letters worried some people in the university concerned that entering a commercial environment would debase the institution's reputation. Situated next door to the Lakeshore Dental Care offices and over the GNC nutrition store on the first level, the clinic makes the western wing of the shopping center almost a medical mall. The clinic offers internal medicine, family medicine, and pediatric services. UCSF opened the clinic on this site because it was a good white-collar neighborhood where they could expect a high rate of insured patients. The university directly marketed the new clinic to the neighborhood, held physician open houses to introduce their practitioners to potential patients, and organized the clinic to improve patient experiences. The clinic was a success soon after its opening, drawing new patients into the UCSF healthcare system.[32]

Most people visiting mini-mall or stand-alone clinics are seeking primary care or urgent-care services, but a growing number are undergoing surgical procedures. Surgery is the foundation upon which the modern hospital was constructed. Successful surgical procedures lured first the wealthy, then the middle class into the hospital, which could offer an expanding set of other services. Ambulatory surgery has the potential to change the equation, by becoming a common procedure. One can easily imagine a professional athlete having arthoscopic surgery in the morning and being back on the field later in the day. That story is still fiction, but by 1991 almost 12 million ambulatory surgeries had been completed. By 1994, the number had jumped to 28.3 million surgical and nonsurgical outpatient procedures during 18.8 million ambulatory surgery visits.[33] People undergoing procedures for which one once stayed in the hospital for days, sometimes months, are in at 8:00 a.m. and out by 4:00 p.m. Changes in equipment, technique, and philosophy have brought doctors to the realization that if you don't need all the accoutrements of the hospital, you don't have to operate there. Surgeons are leaving the hospital for separate, less hospital-like quarters.

In 1997, 70 percent of knee arthoscopic surgeries occurred in hospitals, 82 percent of skin lesion removals were performed in doctor's offices, and 50 percent of eyelid defect repairs were conducted in ambulatory surgery centers.[34] The surgical landscape has become more complex, with competing centers battling for patients by offering the latest in options, technology, and convenience. Importantly, though, all these procedures are performed on an outpatient basis. The vast majority of routine eye surgeries no longer mandate any stay in the hospital.

The result has been the rapid rise of independent surgical clinics, from around 200 in 1970 to over 2,500 in 1998, as the newest development in the medical landscape. An unusual example of this trend came when a specialist in a Fairfax (Virginia) shopping mall placed a viewing screen outside the eye surgery, so mall passers-by could watch the surgery.[35] The ambulatory surgicenters are located in a wide range of sites, including older professional buildings, freestanding commercial buildings, mini-malls, and even regional shopping malls. Market forces are playing a greater role as ambulatory surgery expands and as group practices compete with hospitals for patients. Group practices cannot out compete hospitals for complicated surgeries, but most surgeries are now routine procedures, where off-site, less expensive locations offer an important economic advantage.

Los Angeles's Westside Granville Plaza, designed and built by Richard Donahue in 1988, epitomizes the changing medical landscape. The Plaza is a two-story concrete mini-mall located in the middle of a block along Wilshire Boulevard in the city's wealthy Westside. Its two wings are joined by a center bridge that also serves as the entrance to the mall's underground parking. Its tenants include several restaurants, a photocopy business, and several small businesses. On the upper floor of the eastern wing, a chiropractor and a surgical clinic have offices. The surgical clinic sits just above the photocopying shop. In one way, the mini-mall reconstructs the old Main Street configuration, with the professional offices above the retailers. However, as the Plaza's sign suggests, the clinics are no longer separated from the commercial image of the street. Their bold signs compete for attention, their presence signals a relocation, physically and culturally, onto the street. Professional and commercial uses that have long been carefully separated are mixed in an unruly combination.

Outside, the signs shout in the vernacular of the commercial lexicon, while inside healthcare providers offer professional services in settings that try to imitate long-held standards but with a twist. Mini-mall medicine occurs in buildings that are much smaller and more ordinary than those of conventional healthcare facilities. They are especially distinct from the ornate, complex, and often intimidating internal configuration of the modern hospital, in which patients are forced to navigate endless corridors, waiting rooms, and more corridors before being ushered into a small, too often dreary examination room. Along the way, the physician's importance is constantly reinforced by the furnishings, the barriers between patient and doctor, and the waiting. Even in the postmodern facilities, the spacious atriums, homey waiting rooms, and pastel-colored appointment desks only soften the impact of the multiple barriers and repeated instructions. Typically, the patient is still placed in a subordinate role, told in no uncertain terms about the relative importance of their time and effort in relationship to those of the physician.

The mini-mall, though, eliminates many of the barriers and shifts perceptions of importance. The healthcare facility is now competing for attention with familiar commercial entities. The UCLA clinic's big blue-and-gold sign is notable for its similarity to the pie shop's and the bank's signs. Inside, a barrier still usually greets the patient, but it is a single barrier between the patient and the healthcare provider rather than a series of them. The physical layout recalls the older, long-lamented times when the physician worked out of the home. The elaborate configuration is simplified back to the essentials.

Whether this simplification is affecting the patient-doctor relationship needs to be assessed. The mini-mall or shopping center clinic is not a doctor's home. It is a commercial space, so the intimacy that commentators associate with the older style (actually older place) of medicine is not present in the mini-mall. Still, the dynamic is shifting, with consequences still to be fully understood.

Promoting the Nation's Health

Healthcare is a big business. Recent surveys claim healthcare expenditures represent over 15 percent of the nation's domestic national product (DNP). The most visible elements of that business are not just hospitals or surgi-centers, but also mall diet salons, nutrition outlets, and herbal shops. However, as hospitals and other healthcare organizations have realized that the American obsession with health offers new opportunities to attract potential long-term patients, especially families, they have expanded in-house educational and preventive programs into areas of high pedestrian traffic, like the shopping mall. In a growing number of malls, health fairs occur on a regular basis and diagnostic tests such as mammograms and eye exams are provided periodically. The mall as community center serves as a vehicle for health education and promotion, and, as well, for practitioners and institutions to advertise by offering community services.

The Beverly Center is a regional shopping mall located in the heart of the Los Angeles basin a few miles east of Beverly Hills, just west of Wilshire Boulevard's Miracle Mile. Its next-door neighbor is Cedars-Sinai Medical Center, home to cosmetic surgeons to the stars as well as one of the most prestigious hospitals in the world. Cedars-Sinai has recently opened "Picture Your Health" within the Beverly Center. Here, shoppers can receive preliminary diagnostic testing, health education materials, and other health-related information. When the shop gets busy or people want to wait for their results, they are handed beepers and encouraged to go shopping in the center. If the testing suggests a need for further treatment, the staff will arrange for a visit with a Cedars-Sinai physician at the neighboring facilities. In other words, Picture Your Health not only provides shoppers with health information, it also could provide Cedars-Sinai with new clients.

The boundary between healthcare information as a public service and as a marketing tool has blurred with the increasing competition in the healthcare market. Such a synergy between health education and market competition seems to be well established among healthcare organizations. Many hospital or HMO advertisements at first blush look like health promotion pamphlets, and health fairs and free diagnostic services are often tied to informing shoppers, parents, or community members about other services provided by the same organization. Free refrigerator magnets and other give-aways provide easy reminders of important telephone numbers and increase public awareness of programs.

A Fragile and Dynamic Landscape

As with any researchers exploring a new topic, we were enthralled to find a new medical center opening in the Highland–Wilshire mini-mall described above. Unlike many earlier examples, this one was in a wealthier neighborhood, in a newer mini-mall, near a busy commercial street, with neighboring chiropractic and acupuncture clinics. Within a year, the medical clinic was shuttered. Two stores in the same mini-mall had also closed, including the Kinko's copy center, and the shopping plaza's sign was bare. A window was broken and graffiti were visible. The center was an example of the dynamic and fragile nature of the new medical landscape. In the past, the doctor was expected to stay the same for life, and to stay in the same place. Now, change seems to be more likely than stability.

Such change is even more expected among the private clinics popping up along commercial streets in poor neighborhoods. A medical clinic at the corner of the two busy streets in a mobile Latino neighborhood opened and closed within a year. At around the same time, a clinic opened in a mini-mall near the center of the region's African American community. The clinic welcomed Medicare and Medicaid patients and walk-ins. The small clinic is representative of at least a dozen other clinics around the city. Typically, one or two doctors establish a community practice. In earlier years, they would have located their practice in a small office building. Now, they are on an accessible corner close to a large African American neighborhood as well as the expanding Latino community. Will they be able to succeed in such a location? Will the partnership endure, or the rents rise, or the neighborhood demographics shift? All those factors, and others, will influence the stability of the clinic.

The story of a small clinic in an older shopping center located between Washington and Venice Boulevards in Culver City suggests how powerful are the forces of instability. The grocery store in the center seemed less successful than others operated by the chain, and the center was only half occupied. While the grocery store drew regular traffic, the other stores seemed almost somnolent. The clinic was set in a small stand-alone building at the northern end of the parking lot, right on Venice Boulevard. The clinic faced east, at a perpendicular angle to the street. It was not easily noticed nor well advertised. The rest of the building held a copy store, a barber shop, and a real estate business. The clinic, unable to survive in a shopping center in such poor economic straits, had to move. A handwritten sign announced its new location, along another street in a much more visible location.

Both parts of the mini-mall medicine equation are fraught with instability. Mini-malls are often constructed on short credit lines and are very dependent on rentals to stay profitable. Any economic misfortune can put irrevocable stress on the finances of a small center and its developer. When Southern California entered a protracted recession in the early 1990s, mini-mall construction stopped, and several newspaper articles announced the end of the mini-mall. These calls were welcomed by a wide range of urban planners and designers who found the kitsch architecture of the mini-mall an affront and a symbol of urban blight. However, with the return to prosperity in the late 1990s, new centers began opening and old ones to be renovated. Still, as events at the Wilshire shopping center show, tenant stability is not assured even in times of prosperity.

Such stability is particularly fragile in poorer neighborhoods, which are accustomed to uneven healthcare services. In cities like Los Angeles, immigrants have long looked to local healers, rather than weather the burdens associated with trying to access conventional healthcare services. Unfortunately, as press reports have chronicled, the situation sometimes results in inappropriate care by unqualified practitioners. In late 1998, a 60-year-old toy store employee was arrested for illegally practicing dentistry in the back of the store. On March 2, 1999, the *Los Angeles Times* editorialized about unlicensed clinics, reminding readers of an 18-month-old girl who had died after receiving an injection in an unlicensed clinic in Tustin, California, at least the second death in a year in such a facility. The editorial noted for its readers the complicated circumstances: Many Latin American residents were used to going to local pharmacies for injections. "Some immigrants use unauthorized clinics because they are unaware that low-cost care is available or, if they are here illegally, out of fear of calling attention to themselves. Others prefer neighborhood healers who speak their language." The reasons suggest the gulf some residents feel between themselves and the medical system.

The short lives of mini-mall clinics and the illegal practicing of medicine both suggest that the volatility in medical technology, health systems, and insurance plans that has spread to the physical landscape of medicine. Stability of place, like stability of provider or health plan, is uncertain. The commercialization of medicine, and its relocation into a commercialized landscape, reinforce such uncertainty. Mini-malls more frequently change ownership, raise rents, and shift tenants than was the case in the older residential or professional settings. The high rate of turnover that has come to be expected in the commercial environment is surprising when applied to medicine or any other profession, but such is the new medical landscape.

SHOPPING FOR HEALTHCARE

The increasing desirability of commercial locations for healthcare comes at a time when retail developers are eager for attractions, given the mounting competition between malls and alternative shopping venues, especially the Internet. Many shopping centers and mini-malls in Los Angeles, and elsewhere nationally, are struggling to maintain full occupancy. Many shopping centers have aged, and the communities surrounding them have declined. In Culver City, home of Sony Pictures, Washington Boulevard is dotted with empty retail spaces, and the main shopping center in western downtown is only half occupied. Small stores that prospered in the shopping districts of the 1920s, 1950s, even 1970s, cannot compete with mass merchandisers, outlet malls, and bargain stores.

Medical clinics, which could not have competed with the profits of commercial tenants in the shopping centers' heyday, are attractive potential tenants today. As one Florida leasing agent noted: "Medical groups make good tenants because they're stable and pay their rent on time. . . . Some come to us after they check first-floor rents in their medical-office building and discover that ours are comparable or lower. Besides, we offer more traffic, more exposure, and more convenient parking." He reported that each of the seventeen centers he managed had a medical tenant.[36] One Minnesota HMO has satellite clinics in four malls, including the Mall of America. Especially in the South and West, where mini-mall, strip mall, and even mega-mall construction has produced a glut of available retail space, rental prices are low enough to compete with freestanding medical office buildings.

The healthcare satellites serve a dual purpose. First, they relieve congestion in hospitals and medical centers, which have grown to be medical workshops serving many needs. At the hospital, ambulatory care patients mingle with inpatients, inpatient visitors, medical students, researchers, and the enormous staff. At a satellite center, where well-baby visits and treatment of minor illnesses are the most common services, there are no inpatients and the number and assortment of staff are minimal. Second, the satellite clinics serve as a referral network, sending the more serious, more desirable patients to the medical center. Seen periodically by the primary care staff of the satellite, if a person develops a serious illness necessitating hospitalization, surgery, or a battery of tests, then those will almost assuredly be completed at the home center. Having satellite facilities allows a large medical center to shuttle less-ill patients into more convenient and less costly space and to reserve the medical center for more appropriate and costly procedures.

Ultimately, mini-mall medicine is still in formation. The clinics might be the forerunners of ever more commercialized healthcare, in which physicians and other personnel would become employees of large retail-like chains offering low-cost, low-quality healthcare. Or, these community or neighborhood satellites could be the foundation stones of a new decentralized system of care that would offer accessible primary care to families and individuals, who would then be sent to community hospitals or regional medical centers for more sophisticated and specialized care. In either case, the mini-mall clinics are part of a dynamic medical landscape.

From the dental offices in the local shopping center and the "doc-in-a-box" in the mini-mall to the optometrist's shop in the regional shopping center, these decentralized healthcare facilities are reshaping our experience and perception of healthcare. The flashy signs, the banners that welcome new clients to the mini-mall acupuncture office, and the discounts offered by the dentist at the small shopping center are not just reflections of the changes, but manifestations of them. Medicine may no longer seem as distant for the patient who parks in front of the GNC store to go to the UCSF clinic. The doctor-patient relationship may no longer seem as one-sided to a person who visits a physician in a mini-mall along a commercial street rather than in a large, forbidding downtown edifice. A patient may be emboldened to hold a conversation with a physician if the internal layout of the clinic is less intimidating. Changes in the location of healthcare facilities alter perceptions of medicine, which in turn reinforce the other institutional shifts occurring in healthcare.

EPILOGUE /   Orchestrating Healthcare

The new healthcare system will be ever more likely to incorporate spaces that violate the perceived boundaries of a century ago. The shopping mall emerged as one model for rethinking hospital design because it was more integrated and accessible, which made it more familiar for consumers. Medicine moved to the mini-mall as a logical extension of changing medical practice and increasing market competition. In a perverse irony, America's most prestigious profession utilized one of the culture's least exalted built forms to reorder its relationship with its clientele. Whether infusing the hospital with elements of the mall or transferring pieces of the hospital to the mall and mini-mall, architects and managers have transformed previously staid institutional designs into something much more approachable and have made their services more convenient.

The consequences of these changes are not yet clear. The many risks of commercialism are a serious concern. Medicine has successfully presented itself as a sacred art of great social benefit that is ethically separate from the marketplace. Lowering the boundaries between medical practice and ordinary commercial activities by merging them in the mall may adversely affect people's perceptions of healthcare provision and negatively affect medical practitioners. Efforts to regulate managed care organizations, hospital systems, and other institutional innovations stem from such fears. Physicians and other practitioners continue to worry that relocating and resituating their activities will subject them to new commercial pressures that will be detrimental to their professional activities.

Exemplary of these fears is the continuing attitude toward alternative practitioners. Alternative therapy practitioners have long resided in the commercial realm. While being in these locations familiarized people with their services, it has done little to increase the status of those professionals. Even as America experiences a renaissance in the public's acceptance of complementary medical approaches, their location actually reinforces for many the differences between alternative therapists and "regular" practitioners. Commentators fear that movement of conventional medicine into the street-level retail settings where alternative medicine has resided will cast similar doubts on its practitioners. In addition, they fear that, as a product of this relocation and redesigning of healthcare provision, people will receive lower-quality care, that even greater disparities will develop between haves and have-nots, and that American medicine might undergo a general deterioration.

However, blending medicine and mall may not turn out so badly. It may not produce a crisis but actually create an opportunity for improvement. People may continue to hold medical practitioners in great esteem while finding that they can more conveniently and comfortably access the healthcare system. Or, practitioners may lose status, but healthcare practitioners' communication and compassion may improve. Or, the system may adapt to these location and design changes without noticeable impact on the practice and profession of medicine. The answers simply are not known yet.

An Integrated System

More radically, a new paradigm for thinking about healthcare, and its future might emerge from the current turmoil. The fragmentation and chaos associated with the marketplace may drive participants in the current system to move toward a more effectively designed system. In healthcare, the various pieces of the system are rarely considered in an integrated manner. The long-term facilities are only vaguely connected to hospices, while ambulatory surgery facilities are typically not linked to hospital surgical units. Few practitioners, designers, or commentators look at the system as a whole.

Healthcare analysts are beginning to argue that such an attitude is myopic. Wanda Jones, a healthcare consultant, has noted the exciting opportunities that a fully integrated system would offer architects, as well as the patients that used such facilities. She points out that architects "can help their clients to design delivery systems, not just hospitals; community services networks, not just campuses; and new patient-focused operating systems, not just sets of rooms and spaces for equipment."[1] Her comment is a recognition that the system is made up of many pieces, which are constantly competing with each other, both within a category like hospitals, and also between categories, such as the battle for eye patients between group practices and hospital staffs.

In the commercial realm, elaborate typologies have been developed to portray the entire retail network. The individual retailer in an independent shop is at the foundation of the hierarchy, followed by independently owned stores in strip commercial developments, neighborhood and community shopping centers (including mini-malls), regional shopping malls, and finally, mega-malls. Specialty retail centers, such as outlets, can fit into several categories depending upon their size and location. This hierarchy is only an ideal, and it does not account for all the retail activities in the system. And, the individual units do not always keep their place in the hierarchy; for instance, mini-malls now compete with mega-malls to house certain services. However, the hierarchy provides a systematic perspective that is easily lost when the analyst examines one part of the system, as so often happens with healthcare.

Healthcare has a similar hierarchy: individual practitioners, group practices, hospitals, medical centers with specialty units such as ambulatory surgery and primary care clinics. These elements have specialized roles while also interacting. They also have a geographical hierarchy of service. Individual practitioners usually serve a relatively limited area, while medical centers draw from a whole region, state, or nation. Similarly, a greater range of specialized services is available as one rises in the hierarchy. As with the ideal shopping system, the hierarchy is no longer (if it ever was) static, since group practices may offer some specialties that larger medical centers do not.

Systems combining these elements are emerging, at least organizationally if not in the revolutionary architectural design that Wanda Jones desires. Around the country, alliances between hospitals, clinics, skilled nursing facilities, and individual practitioners are becoming increasingly common under managed care. Some, such as that which joins the Dartmouth-Hitchcock Medical Center, the Lahey Hitchcock Clinic, and the Hitchcock Alliance, range across large areas; the facilities in the system stretch from Newport, Vermont, to Waltham, Massachusetts, and from Dover, Maine, to Rutland, Vermont. This network reflects the enormous pressure on physicians to join groups, on groups to associate with hospitals and clinics, and on hospitals and clinics to associate with larger, more viable healthcare systems. Such alliances of providers, clinics, and hospitals provide the basis for greater integration, even as they create fears of monopoly and gaps in service networks.

These broader service networks, whether in the rural outback of northern New England or along the boulevards of Los Angeles, offer the basis for fulfilling long-held hopes that an integrated system of care could be created. A recent article in *Hospital and Health Networks* was titled, "Build It, and They Might Come." The "It" of the title was a "seamless system of care" for the chronically ill which merged home healthcare, hospital care, housing, long-term care, hospice programs, and behavioral health activities. The need for such a system is broadly recognized. As one advocate of a coordinated healthcare system asserts, "We are a system, and now we have to start acting like one."[2] Most commentators agree, though, that a system will not be easily constructed, given the competition among healthcare companies, the disparate nature of patient payment sources, the lack of connections between the various elements of the system, and the absence of a facilitator to manage a patient's relationship with each part of the system.

Shifting the place of medicine out of the isolated professional building into the commercial property may reinforce the need and desirability of integration. As medicine sheds the veil of ignorance regarding the commercial nature of its industry, some long-held prohibitions against thinking in terms that benefit the consumer may fall away. Regina Herzlinger's example of the eyecare industry is instructive here. Removing legal prohibitions that limited the consumer's right to shop for glasses and contacts has revolutionized the industry, invigorated changes in the styles and types of eyewear that are available, all without the disasters predicted by opponents. Obviously, other elements of the healthcare system are less easily opened to consumer choice. Again, obviously, limits are always going to exist on how far such a trend can proceed. Still, if buildings are constructed to welcome patients, in locations that are chosen for their convenience for patients, with staffs that are truly patient focused, a new healthcare environment may emerge.

The new system, though, does not have to depend on a few healthcare mega-companies offering every service in their designated markets. Healthcare consultant Christopher Press has argued that shopping malls offer more than a new location for medical services. He suggests that malls, along with airports, actually offer an organizational paradigm that would allow a more integrated system to emerge.[3] He notes that for much of the twentieth century, the hospital has been organized on the factory model. Two variants of the factory model have been attempted. Using the auto industry as the archetype, some theorists argued that hospitals should have a vertical integration, to "create a health care behemoth that could prevent disease, treat disease in any venue and finance the entire transaction." Others asserted that integration is less important than specialization. They also depended on the factory model, but they rejected vertical integration as too unwieldy and impractical. They tried to master a smaller, focused field of technology. Press responds that both approaches ill-fit the healthcare industry. "Hospitals don't manufacture anything, the analogy is malignantly unsuitable." The manufacturing model implies linear processes, economies of scale, and the ability to build something from disparate parts and to store the final product for eventual sale. Patients, conversely, act in nonlinear fashion, offer few economies of scale, are prepackaged as a complex integrated organism, and healthcare offers many services that cannot be stored.

In suggesting that hospitals and other healthcare organizations look to airports and shopping malls for new ways to organize their activities, Press finds in these organizations a focus on orchestration, not manufacturing. These entities do not *provide* all the services themselves, but they orchestrate the spaces in which the various services are provided. "Shopping malls would never attempt to 'be' all the stores within their walls, from Victoria's Secret to Brooks Brothers." Orchestrators sponsor, providing a "functional, economical infrastructure" in which they convene others to perform services. Hospitals could emulate such orchestration by relying on clinical outsourcing, delegating clinical activities and departments to specialist organizations, and attracting specialists to provide services within the infrastructure the hospital controls. Yes, hospitals would have to give up some control. Still, just as the mall offers a new paradigm for designing accessible, familiar spaces that patients can use more comfortably, it suggests a new way of imagining the organization of individual and systemwide changes in healthcare.

A Nice Story, but Will Any of It Matter in a Virtual World?

Christopher Press's suggestion comes with the qualification that shifting from a factory model to one based on the orchestration of the airport or shopping mall would not be equally appropriate for all healthcare organizations. Similarly, not all future hospitals should or will mimic shopping malls, hotels, or residences. Nor will all services be dispersed into mini-malls. The healthcare industry is so varied and complex that to suggest any one future alternative pathway would be foolish.

A competing vision suggests that the system is going to continue to fragment. The three essays in this volume chronicle the evolution of the medical landscape from the doctor's and patient's home to sparsely furnished mini-mall clinics, plush ambulatory care buildings, and high-tech specialized treatment facilities. A new landscape is emerging. That new landscape is more accessible but continues to reflect economic disparities characteristic of its predecessor. It evidences a renewed attempt to balance care and cure, yet it offers no assurance that medicine will not continue to react to illness rather than try to prevent it. And it relocates medicine into a more commercial space, which might only increase pressures to cut corners and offer bite-sized medicine. The landscape is still forming in the tumult of biomedical innovations, financial revolutions, and social revisions of the last twenty years. These essays are not predictive, just suggestive of how those fundamental changes in medical practice, healthcare financing, and urban and suburban development have evolved and are currently shifting.

Recently, emerging technologies and changing retail trends have raised cautionary flags about where the evolution of healthcare provision is headed. One potentially very disruptive trend is the Internet's impact on healthcare provision. Seeking medical advice in popular literature is nothing new. Health advice books have been published for centuries. In times of great medical advances or controversies, such as the 1840s, 1890s, and 1980s, an avalanche of such publications appeared as writers tried to interpret the implications for their readers. Popular magazines have been offering health news and medical advice since their inception roughly 150 years ago. Newspapers have long carried stories on recent advances in medicine and advertisements offering a variety of healthcare solutions—some conventional, some not. Indeed, in recent decades, medical journals, to heighten the impact of their articles, have developed policies for ensuring that the articles are not discussed in the press prior to publication and that the journal titles are mentioned prominently when information from the articles is published.

That the Internet is simply an extension of these previous sources is doubtful. It offers an immediacy and chance for dialogue that the other media do not. The Internet is such a recent invention, and in such disarray, that any attempts at understanding its impact on our lives are bound to prove shortsighted. However, the Internet is rapidly becoming an extraordinary vehicle for reaching a growing number of people in America, as well as internationally. While it suffers the same inequality of accessibility born of economic disparity that plagues other aspects of the healthcare industry, a growing number of computer stations are available in public places, such as libraries, and evolving technologies promise that anyone with a television will in the future have access to the Internet. Healthcare advice is already widely offered on the Internet, although the sources vary dramatically in reliability. Government agencies, such as the Centers for Disease Control and Prevention, maintain sites that display a plethora of information on topics ranging from HIV/AIDS to travel health. Many hospitals and healthcare organizations have sites where they dispense information about health education and disease prevention, as well as on every type of disease and treatment. The depth and breadth of the data are quite remarkable.

So, the promise of the Internet is that it will lower the expertise disparity between patient and provider by making available to patients many of the sources read by practitioners. Better informed patients may be less passive and more assertive in participating in their care. The Internet may even offer new and efficient avenues for the provision of healthcare. "Distance medicine," in which providers treat patients who are in another location, is already being practiced on-line as well as through other media, such as teleconferencing. The possibilities seem limitless given the technical capability to send patient records through email, share test results on dual computer screens, and conduct face-to-face video dialogues. The possibilities, of course, are not actually unlimited. Surgery will still require a real patient, as will invasive tests and other interventions. Even lesser diagnostic and treatment procedures, such as physical examinations, seem better completed with both parties in the same room.

Instead of empowering the patient, the technology may further alienate the patient from the caregiver. Even though medical schools now have students interact with real patients as quickly as possible, some doctors have expressed the fear that the new generation of physicians cannot use a stethoscope properly and do not touch patients enough.[4] They have been trained to rely on tests, such as blood work-ups, for diagnosis and decisions about treatment. Critics worry that a lack of sensitivity to other kinds of bodily signals will lead some clinicians to miss important indicators of illness. Further, these methodological changes are symbolic of an emotional distancing of clinicians from their patients, a separation that has been aggravated by managed care. Even as patients fight to limit the effects of managed care and to modify the sterility of mid-century medicine, the Internet may serve to draw physicians farther away from patients physically and to force them to practice an electronic medicine that is only a new type of machine medicine. The balance between technology and touch may be even more difficult to maintain in this environment.

Healthcare providers realize the current system's limitations. They share patients' concerns about the system and wish to maintain contact with patients. However, will the continuing obsession with containing cost force doctors to sit in front of video screens to "see" patients? We hope not. Or, will a system evolve in which healthcare providers and consumers are able to overcome the effects of competition to develop an effective, humane, accessible, and high-quality healthcare system? Will it be a system that is part of the commercial world, but one that continues to value ethical professional practices? The hospital model as it evolved between 1870 and 1970 has been and will continue to be transformed by changes in medical practice and healthcare financing, and by consumer demands for humane, accessible, and familiar medical spaces. Medicine is moving into a new era. The healthcare landscape is going to be varied and diverse, dynamic and rapidly evolving.

Notes

Prologue: The Evolving Architecture of Healthcare

1. Ira G. Zepp, Jr., *The New Religious Image of Urban America: Shopping Malls as Ceremonial Centers*, 2nd ed. (Boulder: University Press of Colorado, 1997), p. 10.

2. "Continuum of Care," *Hospitals and Health Networks* 69, no. 18 (1995), p. 14.

3. Paul Groth, "Frameworks for Cultural Landscape Study," in Paul Groth and Todd Bressi, eds., *Understanding Ordinary Landscapes* (New Haven: Yale University Press, 1997), p. 1.

4. George Rosen, "The Hospital: Historical Sociology of a Community Institution," in Eliot Freidson, ed., *The Hospital in Modern Society* (New York: Free Press of Glencoe, 1963), p. 2.

5. W. G. Wylie, *Hospitals: Their History, Organization, and Construction*, Boylston Prize Essay of Harvard University for 1876 (New York: D. Appleton, 1877), p. 134.

6. William Ludlow, "Why Not Homelike Hospitals" (condensed version of article originally published in *Hospital Management*), *Literary Digest* 60 (January 18, 1919), p. 19.

7. Eli Ginzberg, *Tomorrow's Hospitals: A Look to the Twenty-First Century* (New Haven: Yale University Press, 1996), pp. 6–7.

8. H. Ralph Hawkins, "Health Care Malls," *Journal of Health Care Interior Design* 2 (1990), pp. 137–40.

9. Quoted in Stephen Verderber and David J. Fine, *Healthcare Architecture in an Era of Radical Transformation* (New Haven: Yale University Press, 2000), p. 193.

10. Rosen, "The Hospital," p. 2.

11. James Howard Kunstler, *Home From Nowhere: Remaking Our Everyday World for the Twentieth Century* (New York: Simon & Schuster, 1996), quote on p. 59; for his broader view of the car culture, see pp. 58–80.

12. Kenneth Jackson, *Crabgrass Frontier: The Suburbanization of the United States* (New York: Oxford University Press, 1985), pp. 246–71.

13. Regina E. Herzlinger, *Market-Driven Healthcare: Who Wins, Who Loses in the Transformation of America's Largest Service Industry* (Reading, Mass.: Addison-Wesley, 1997), pp. 19, 16, 17–45.

One: The Medical Workshop

1. Helen Eastman Martin, *The History of the Los Angeles County Hospital (1878–1968) and the Los Angeles County–University of Southern California Medical Center (1968–1978)* (Los Angeles: University of Southern California Press, 1979), esp. pp. 98–121.

2. Morris Vogel, "The Transformation of the American Hospital," in Susan Reverby and David Rosner, eds., *Healthcare in America: Essays in Social History* (Philadelphia: Temple University Press, 1979), p. 106.

3. Robert F. Dalzell, Jr., and Lee Baldwin Dalzell, *George Washington's Mount Vernon: At Home in Revolutionary America* (New York: Oxford University Press, 1998), p. 224.

4. Edward F. Stevens, *The American Hospital of the Twentieth Century* (New York: Architectural Record Company, 1921), pp. 358–65.

5. The dates for the hospital's completion are from Thomas G. Morton and Frank Woodbury, *The History of the Pennsylvania Hospital, 1751–1895* (Philadelphia: Times Printing House, 1897), pp. 39, 78, and 80. A photograph of the John Kinsey house as a hospital can be seen in Ann Novotny and Carter Smith, *Images of Healing: A Portfolio of American Medical and Pharmaceutical Practice in the Eighteenth, Nineteenth, and Twentieth Centuries* (New York: Macmillan, 1980), p. 17. The surroundings are described in, William H. Williams, *America's First Hospital: The Pennsylvania Hospital, 1751–1941* (Wayne, Pa.: Haverford House, 1976), pp. 21–24.

6. J. M. Toner, "Statistics of Regular Medical Associations and Hospitals of the United States," *Transactions of the American Medical Association* 24 (1873), pp. 285–333. Toner's study lists 178 hospitals, but almost 50 of them were exclusively for the mentally ill, so 128 is Toner's count of general hospitals. This figure clearly undercounts the nation's hospitals. For instance, Los Angeles is not listed as having a hospital, but by 1873, the city had two, Sister's and the French Hospital.

7. John Shaw Billings, "Notes on Hospital Construction," *Public Health Reports and Papers of the American Public Health Association Meeting, 1874–75,* (New York: Hurd & Houghton, 1876), pp. 385–88.

8. John Green, *City Hospitals* (Boston: Little Brown, 1861), p. 14.

9. Quoted in Charles E. Rosenberg *The Care of Strangers: The Rise of America's Hospital System* (New York: Basic Books, 1987), p. 52.

10. W. G. Wylie, *Hospitals: Their History, Organization, and Construction*, Boyl-

ston Prize Essay of Harvard University for 1876 (New York: D. Appleton, 1877), pp. 57–58, 187, 58–59.

11. Robert Morris, *Fifty Years a Surgeon* (New York: E. P. Dutton, 1938).

12. Rosemary Stevens, *In Sickness and In Health: American Hospitals in the Twentieth Century* (New York: Basic Books, 1989), p. 24.

13. Christine Stevenson, "Medicine and Architecture," in W. F. Bynum and Roy Porter, eds., *Companion Encyclopedia of the History of Medicine,* vol. 2 (London: Routledge, 1993), p. 1510.

14. Caroline Hannaway, "Environment and Miasmata," in W. F. Bynum and Roy Porter, eds., *Companion Encyclopedia of the History of Medicine,* vol. 1 (London: Routledge, 1993), p. 295.

15. Quoted in Judith Walzer Leavitt and Ronald Numbers, *Sickness and Health in America* (Madison: University of Wisconsin Press, 1978), p. 3.

16. John M. Woodworth, "Hospitals and Their Construction: The Principles Which Should Govern in the Location, Design, Material, General Management, and Duration of Use of Hospitals," *Public Health Reports and Papers of the American Public Health Association Meeting, 1874–75* (New York: Hurd & Houghton, 1876), pp. 389–90.

17. Florence Nightingale, quoted in Nikolaus Pevsner, *A History of Building Types* (Princeton, N.J.: Princeton University Press, 1976), p. 155.

18. For general discussions of the pavilion hospital, see Jeremy Taylor, *The Architect and the Pavilion Hospital: Dialogue and Design Creativity in England, 1850–1914* (London: Leicester University Press, 1997) and John D. Thompson and Grace Goldin, *The Hospital: A Social and Architectural History* (New Haven: Yale University Press, 1975), pp. 208–9. J. Green, *City Hospitals* mentions pavilions as a response to miasmias (pp. 25–38).

19. Lindsay Prior, "The Architecture of the Hospital: A Study of Spatial Organization and Medical Knowledge," *British Journal of Sociology* 39, no. 1 (March 1988), p. 94.

20. W. Gilman Thompson, "Modern Hospital Construction," *American Journal of Medical Science* 49, no. 12 (1906), pp. 998–99.

21. Christian Holmes, *The Planning of a Modern Hospital: An Address Delivered Before the Department of Nursing and Health, Teacher's College, Columbia University, February 21, 1911* (Detroit: National Hospital Record Publishing, 1911), p. 9.

22. E. Stevens, *The American Hospital of the Twentieth Century,* pp. 16–17.

23. William J. Horvath and Raymond J. Cristina, *West Penn Heritage: 125 Years, 1848–1973* (privately published, 1973).

24. Dell Upton, *Architecture in the United States* (New York: Oxford University Press, 1998), p. 157.

25. Richard H. Shryock, *The Unique Influence of the Johns Hopkins University on American Medicine* (Copenhagen: Ejnar Munksgaard, 1953).

26. Rosenberg, *Care of Strangers*, pp. 212–36.

27. Abraham Flexner, *Medical Education in the United States and Canada* (New York: Carnegie Foundation, 1910); also see, Kenneth M. Ludmerer, *Learning to Heal: The Development of American Medical Education* (New York: Basic Books, 1985).

28. Ephraim McDowell, "Three Cases of Extirpation of Diseased Ovaria," in, Gert H. Brieger, ed., *Medical America in the Nineteenth Century* (Baltimore: Johns Hopkins Press, 1972), pp. 166–68.

29. Paul Starr, *The Social Transformation of American Medicine: The Rise of a Sovereign Profession and the Making of a Vast Industry* (New York: Basic Books, 1982), p. 157.

30. No general history of children's hospitals has been written. The most recent effort to discuss their histories is Janet Golden, ed., *Infant Asylums and Children's Hospitals: Medical Dilemmas and Developments, 1850–1920, An Anthology of Sources* (New York: Garland, 1989).

31. Mary Rogers, "Children's Hospitals in America," in J. S. Billings and H. M. Hurd, eds., *Hospitals, Dispensaries, and Nursing: Papers and Discussions in the International Congress of Charities, Correction and Philanthropy, Section III, Chicago, June 12th to 17th, 1893* (Baltimore: Johns Hopkins Press, 1894), pp. 373–74.

32. Jeffrey P. Brosco, "Policy and Poverty: Child and Community Health in Philadelphia, 1900–1930," *Archives of Pediatrics and Adolescent Medicine* 149, no. 12 (December 1995), p. 1382.

33. E. Stevens, *The American Hospital of the Twentieth Century*, p. 149.

34. Rogers, "Children's Hospitals in America," p. 378.

35. R. Stevens, *In Sickness and In Health*, pp. 230–31, 24, 333, 259.

36. Eli Ginzberg, *The Road to Reform: The Future of Healthcare in America* (New York: Free Press, 1994), pp. 67–75.

37. Rosenberg, *Care of Strangers*, pp. 244–45.

38. J. Corse quoted in Robert Somer and Robert Dewar "The Physical Environment of the Ward," in Eliot Freidson, *The Hospital in Modern Society* (New York: Free Press of Glencoe, 1963), p. 321.

39. Winfred Rhoades, "Can Hospitals Be Humane?" *The Survey* 54 (June 1925), pp. 303–4, 314.

40. Janet Golden and Charles E. Rosenberg, *Pictures of Health: A Photographic History of Healthcare in Philadelphia, 1860–1945* (Philadelphia: University of Pennsylvania Press, 1991).

41. For a discussion of these nursing units, see Isadore Rosenfield, *Hospitals: Integrated Design* (New York: Progressive Architecture Library, 1947), pp. 49–67.

42. William Ludlow, "Why Not Homelike Hospitals?" *Literary Digest* 60 (January 18, 1919), p. 19; article by A. Bacon, in *Hospital Management* (Chicago, 1919), reprinted as "A Hospital Like a Hotel" in *Literary Digest* 61 (June 21, 1919), pp. 111–15.

43. Thompson and Goldin, *The Hospital*, pp. 207–25.

44. Michael Bobrow, "The Evolution of Nursing Space Planning for Efficient Operation," *Architectural Record* (1971).

45. Charles F. Neergaard et al., "Planning the Small General Hospital," *Architectural Record* (December 1939), p. 77.

46. Quoted in Thompson and Goldin, *The Hospital*, p. 182.

47. Rosenfield, *Hospitals: Integrated Design*, p. 43.

48. Taylor, *The Architect and the Pavilion Hospital*, summarizes the growing literature on hospital architecture. He focuses on English and European works, but he includes most of the relevant American work up to the early twentieth century, pp. 40–71.

49. Annmarie Adams, "Modernism and Medicine: The Hospitals of Stevens and Lee, 1916–1932," *Journal of the Society of Architectural Historians* 58, no. 1 (March 1999), pp. 42–61; on Goldwater, see his groundbreaking article, "Notes on Hospital Planning," which appeared in *The Brickbuilder* in 1912.

50. Adams, "Modernism and Medicine."

51. E. Stevens, *The American Hospital of the Twentieth Century*, p. 2.

52. Jacque B. Norman, "Administrative Aspects of Hospital Design," in, American Institute of Architects, *Hospitals: Convention Seminar Addresses*. (Washington, D.C.: AIA, 1947), p. 45.

53. Walter A. Tompkins, *Cottage Hospital: The First Hundred Years* (Santa Barbara, Calif.: Santa Barbara Cottage Hospital Foundation, 1988).

54. The following discussion depends on Eugene Julius Grow, "The Mary Hitchcock Hospital," *Granite Monthly* (1896), pp. 247–58; Megan McAndrew Cooper, *A History of Mary Hitchcock Memorial Hospital* (published by the hospital, 1994); and pamphlets and ephemera from the "Mary Hitchcock Memorial Vertical File" in the Special Collections of Dartmouth College.

55. Temple Burling, Edith M. Lentz, and Robert N. Wilson, *The Give and Take in Hospitals* (1956), quoted in R. Stevens, *In Sickness and In Health*, p. 231.

56. Ivan Illich, *Medical Nemesis: The Expropriation of Health* (New York: Random House, 1976): esp. pp. 32–34; *Illustrated Stedman's Medical Dictionary*, 24th ed. (Baltimore: Williams & Wilkins, 1982), p. 688.

57. Charles Rosenberg, "Community and Communities: The Evolution of the American Hospital," in Diana Elizabeth Long and Janet Golden, eds., *The American General Hospital: Communities and Social Context* (Ithaca, N.Y.: Cornell University Press, 1989), p. 4.

Two: Humanizing the Hospital

Paragraphs from this chapter also appear in, David Charles Sloane, "Scientific

Paragon to Hospital Mall: The Evolving Design of the Hospital, 1885–1994," *Journal of Architectural Education* 48, no. 2 (November 1994), and David Charles Sloane, "In Search of a Hospitable Hospital," *Dartmouth Medicine* 18, no. 1 (Fall 1993).

1. David Charles Sloane, "In Search of a Hospitable Hospital," *Dartmouth Medicine* 18, no. 1 (Fall 1993), pp. 23–31; Rosemary Lunardini, "A New England Medical Village," *Dartmouth Medicine* 16, no. 1 (Fall 1991), pp. 28–33; John Gregerson, "Medical Center Adds Human Touch to Healthcare," *Building Design and Construction* (August 1992), pp. 24–29; and W. Mason Smith and Frederick W. Nothnagel, "Case Study: Dartmouth Hitchcock Medical Center" (for Shepley Bulfinch Richardson and Abbott, Boston, ca. 1990); and materials in the Dartmouth College Special Collections.

2. Thanks to Annelise Orleck and Alexis Jetter for this observation.

3. Mitchel Green, "American Healthcare Design: Search for a New Image," *a+u* 201 (1987), p. 104.

4. Stephen Verderber and David J. Fine, *Healthcare Architecture in an Era of Radical Transformation* (New Haven: Yale University Press, 2000), p. 86.

5. Julie Marquis, "UCLA Looks to Future in Reshaping Medical Complex," *Los Angeles Times* (January 19, 1999), p. 19.

6. Thomas Bender, in "City Life," *Los Angeles Times* (December 22, 1996); Kenneth Helphand, "McUrbia: The 1950s and the Birth of the Contemporary American Landscape," *Places* 5, no. 2 (1988), pp. 40–49.

7. Richard Longstreth, *City Center to Regional Mall: Architecture, the Automobile, and Retailing in Los Angeles, 1920–1950* (Cambridge, Mass: MIT Press, 1997); Greg Hise, *Magnetic Los Angeles: Planning the Twentieth-Century Metropolis* (Baltimore: Johns Hopkins University Press, 1997).

8. Meredith Clausen, "Shopping Centers," in J. Wilkes, ed., *Encyclopedia of Architecture: Design, Engineering, and Construction*, 4 vols. (New York: John Wiley & Sons, 1989), pp. 406–21.

9. Victor Gruenbaum (later Gruen) and Elsie Krummech, "New Buildings for 194x: Shopping Center," *Architectural Forum* 78, no. 5 (May 1943), pp. 101–3.

10. Clausen, "Shopping Centers." Also see, Victor Gruen, *The Heart of Our Cities, The Urban Crisis: Diagnosis and Cure* (New York: Simon & Schuster, 1964).

11. Ira G. Zepp, Jr., *The New Religious Image of Urban America: Shopping Malls as Ceremonial Centers*, 2nd ed. (Boulder: University Press of Colorado, 1997).

12. The examples from Baptist Outpatient Center in Jacksonville and St. Louis Children's Hospital / West County Satellite Health Center are taken from Richard L. Miller and Earl S. Swensson, *New Directions in Hospital and Healthcare Facility Design* (New York: McGraw-Hill, 1995); all the other examples are from Verderber and Fine, *Healthcare Architecture in an Era of Radical Transformation*. Also see, David C. Sloane, "Scientific Paragon to Hospital Mall: The Evolving Design of the Hos-

pital, 1885–1994," *Journal of Architectural Education* 48, no. 2 (November 1994), pp. 82–98.

13. Verderber and Fine, *Healthcare Architecture in an Era of Radical Transformation*, pp. 86–88.

14. Sloane, "Scientific Paragon to Hospital Mall," pp. 82–98.

15. A.O.D. [Andrea Oppenheimer Dean], "Emergency Unit Puts a Welcoming Face on a Hospital," *Architecture* 75, no. 4 (April 1986), p. 65.

16. Donald McKahan, "The Healing Environment of the Future," *Healthcare Forum* (May–June 1990), p. 37.

17. A.O.D., "Emergency Unit Puts a Welcoming Face on a Hospital," p. 64.

18. Miller and Swensson, *New Directions in Hospital and Healthcare Facility Design*, p. 22.

19. Celebration Health and St. John's promotional materials; Bernadette Peters, "A Hospital Like Home," *Architecture South* 3, no. 1 (1996); and Andrea Oppenheimer Dean, "Sharon Hospital, Sharon, Connecticut," *Architectural Record* 185, no. 5 (May 1997), p. 174–76.

20. Andrea Oppenheimer Dean, "Alta Bates Cancer Center, Berkeley, California," *Architectural Record* 185, no. 5 (May 1997), p. 182–86.

21. John Shaw Billings, "Notes on Hospital Construction," *Public Health Reports and Papers of the American Public Health Association Meeting, 1874–75* (New York: Hurd & Houghton, 1876); "Architectural Record's Building Types Study #116: Notes on Hospital Planning," *Architectural Record* 101 (August 1946).

22. William Ludlow, "Why Not Homelike Hospitals?" (condensed version of article originally published in *Hospital Management* in 1918), *Literary Digest* 60 (January 18, 1919), p. 19.

23. George Rosen, "The Hospital: Historical Sociology of a Community Institution," in Eliot Freidson, ed., *The Hospital in Modern Society* (New York: Free Press of Glencoe, 1963).

24. N. R. G., "Redesigning Healthcare," *Architecture* (April 1986), pp. 68–70.

25. Edward F. Stevens, *The American Hospital of the Twentieth Century* (New York: Architectural Record Company, 1921), p. 126.

26. Isadore Rosenfield, *Hospitals: Integrated Design* (New York: Reinhold, 1947), pp. 125–26.

27. John Morton, "Fathers in the Delivery Room," *Bulletin of the Los Angeles County Medical Association* 94 (October 15, 1964), p. 20. The emphasis is in the original.

28. Margaret Gaskie, "Making Special Care Special," *Architectural Record* (June 1990), pp. 98–101.

29. Linheim quote from N. R. G., "Redesigning Healthcare," p. 70; York quote from Troy Segal, "Hospitals You May Hate to Leave," *Business Week* (June 8, 1990), p. 146.

30. For an overview of the history of organized ambulatory care, see Emil F. Pascarelli, ed., *Hospital-Based Ambulatory Care* (Norwalk, Conn.: Appleton-Century-Crofts, 1982), and Milton I. Roemer, *Ambulatory Health Services in America: Past, Present, and Future* (Rockville, Md.: Aspen, 1981).

31. Information on the dispensary comes from Charles E. Rosenberg, *The Care of Strangers: The Rise of America's Hospital System* (New York: Basic Books, 1987); Michael M. Davis and Andrew R. Warner, *Dispensaries: Their Management and Development* (New York: Macmillan, 1918); and Michael M. Davis, *Clinics, Hospitals and Health Centers* (New York: Harper & Brothers, 1927).

32. Davis, *Clinics, Hospitals and Health Centers*; E. Stevens, *The American Hospital of the Twentieth Century*, pp. 227–42.

33. E. Stevens, *The American Hospital of the Twentieth Century*, p. 230; Rosenberg, *The Care of Strangers*, pp. 172–74; E. Stevens, *The American Hospital of the Twentieth Century*, p. 234.

34. E. Stevens, *The American Hospital of the Twentieth Century*, p. 234.

35. Charles F. Neergaard et al., "Planning the Small General Hospital," *Architectural Record* 86 (December 1939), p. 78; E. H. L. Corwin, *The American Hospital* (New York: The Commonwealth Fund, 1946), p. 164.

36. Emerson Goble, "Hospitals: Building Type Study #158: St. Clare's Hospital, Schenectady, New York," *Architectural Record* 107 (1950), pp. 121–22.

37. Roemer, *Ambulatory Health Services in America*, pp. 1–29, 47–62; Jerry Alan Solon, "Outpatient Care: A Term in Search of a Concept," *Hospitals* 39, no. 6 (March 16, 1965), pp. 61–65. Also see, E. Richard Weinerman, "Changing Patterns in Medical Care: Their Implications for Ambulatory Services," *Hospitals* 39, no. 24 (December 16, 1965), pp. 67–74, 108.

38. American Hospital Association, *Hospital Statistics* (Chicago: AHA, 1999), p. 2.

39. Clifford A. Pearson, "Building Types Study #749: Healthcare Facilities: Whither the Hospital?" *Architectural Record* (May 1997), p. 165.

40. Jain Malkin, "Creating Excellence in Health Care Design," *Journal of Health Care Interior Design* 3 (1991), p. 28. Also see her excellent discussion of these issues in Jain Malkin, *Hospital Interior Architecture: Creating Healing Environments for Special Patient Populations* (New York: Van Nostrand Reinhold, 1992).

41. Clifford A. Pearson, "Outpatient Services Addition," *Architectural Record* 182, no. 5 (1994), pp. 100–103.

42. Malkin, "Creating Excellence in Healthcare Design," p. 30.

43. Andrea Oppenheimer Dean, "Sharon Hospital," pp. 174–77.

44. Ludlow, "Why Not Homelike Hospitals?" p. 19.

45. Susan Doubilet, "Reassuring Goals," *Progressive Architecture* 8 (1986), p. 80.

46. Margaret Gaskie, "Serious Play," *Architectural Record* 178 (May 1990), p. 96.

47. The web site's address is www.aafpages.org/Stanford.htm.

48. Jane Boone, "Medical Mall Has It All," *Texas Hospitals* (March 1988), pp. 26–28.

49. H. Ralph Hawkins, "Health Care Malls," *Journal of Health Care Interior Design* 2 (1990), pp. 137–40.

50. Ibid.

51. Nita McCann, "Preconstruction of Jackson Medical Mall Well Underway," *Mississippi Business Journal* 18, no. 34 (August 19–25, 1996).

52. Description from Debra Beachy, "Hospital's Opening Will Complete Medical Mall," *Houston Chronicle* (May 7, 1991); quote from Victoria McNamara, "Shopping Mall Hospital First in Country," *Houston Business Journal* 20, no. 35 (January 21, 1991).

53. McKahan, "The Healing Environment of the Future," p. 36.

54. Lucette Lagnado, "What's a Hospital?" *Wall Street Journal* (October 18, 1999), p. R17. Other information on Celebration Health comes from their promotional brochures.

55. Barbara J. Huelat, "Celebration Health Reviewed," *Aesclepius Newsletter of The Center for Health Design* (n.d.), (www.healthdesign.org).

56. Pearson, "Building Types: Whither the Hospital?" p. 165.

57. John Kasson, *Civilizing the Machine: Technology and Republican Values in America, 1776–1900* (New York: Grossman, 1976).

Three: Shopping for Healthcare

Paragraphs from this chapter also appear in, David C. Sloane, "Medicine Moves into the (Mini) Mall," in Paul Groth and Chris Wilson, eds., *J. B. Jackson and American Cultural Landscapes* (Berkeley: University of California Press, 2002).

1. Don Lee, "UC Accused of Plan to Control Patient Care," *Los Angeles Times* (December 10, 1998), p. A15. During an interview on April 7, 1998, Dr. Peter Karpf provided keen insight into UCLA's activities.

2. Berkeley Rice, "Put Your Practice Where Shoppers Throng?" *Medical Economics* 70, no. 2 (1993), p. 138.

3. James H. Kunstler, *The Geography of Nowhere: The Rise and Decline of America's Man-made Landscape* (New York: Touchstone, 1993), p. 21. For an opposing view, see Timothy Davis, "The Miracle Mile Revisited: Recycling, Renovation, and Simulation along the Commercial Strip," in Annmarie Adams and Sally McMurry, eds., *Exploring Everyday Landscapes: Perspectives in Vernacular Architecture*, vol. 7 (Knoxville: University of Tennessee Press, 1997), pp. 93–114.

4. Richard Longstreth, *City Center to Regional Mall: Architecture, the Automobile,*

and Retailing in Los Angeles, 1920–1950 (Cambridge, Mass.: MIT Press, 1997); and his companion volume, *The Drive-in, the Supermarket, and the Transformation of Commercial Space in Los Angeles, 1914–1941* (Cambridge, Mass.: MIT Press, 1999).

5. In California in 1994, approximately eight million residents were uninsured, of which two and one-half million were full-time, year-round employees, according to the *California Healthcare Fact Book, 1999* (Sacramento: Office of Statewide Health Planning and Development, 1999), pp. 10–11.

6. David M. Eisenberg, Roger B. Davis, Susan L. Eitner, Scott Appel, Sonja Wikey, Maria Van Rompay, and Ronald C. Kessler, "Trends in Alternative Medicine Use in the United States, 1990–1997," *JAMA* 280, no. 18 (November 11, 1998), pp. 1571–72. Also see, Terrence Monmaney and Shari Roan, "Hope or Hype? Alternative Medicine Is Edging into the Mainstream, with Californians Leading the Way," *Los Angeles Times* (August 30, 1998), pp. 1, 12.

7. The first quote is from John Brinckerhoff Jackson, "The Future of the Vernacular," in Paul Groth and Todd Bressi, eds., *Understanding Ordinary Landscapes* (New Haven: Yale University Press, 1997), pp. 152–53; the second is from "The Vernacular City," in Helen Horowitz, ed., *Landscapes in Sight: Looking at America* (New Haven: Yale University Press, 1997), p. 238.

8. "Business Building Progress," *American Globe* 6, no. 6 (1909), pp. 1–2.

9. Figures from William G. Rothstein, ed., *Readings in American Health Care: Current Issues in Socio-Historical Perspective* (Madison: University of Wisconsin Press, 1995), pp. 162, 161.

10. David McBride, *Integrating the City of Medicine: Blacks in Philadelphia Healthcare, 1910–1965* (Philadelphia: Temple University Press, 1989), p. 130. Quote from Milton I. Roemer, "Growth of Salaried Physicians," *Hospital Progress* 45, no. 79 (September 1964), in Eugene B. Crawford, Jr., "Annual Administrative Reviews," *Hospitals* 39, no. 7 (April 1965), p. 43.

11. Advertisement, "Designed to Serve the Needs of the Medical Profession," *Los Angeles County Medical Association Bulletin* 94, no. 21 (November 5, 1964), p. 11.

12. Advertisement, "Los Altos Medical Building," *Los Angeles County Medical Association Bulletin* 94, no. 24 (December 3, 1964), p. 38.

13. A broader comment on the changing built environment can be found in Robert Venturi, Denise Scott Brown, and Stephen Izenour, *Learning from Las Vegas* (Cambridge, Mass.: MIT Press, 1977).

14. Jackson, "The Vernacular City," p. 245.

15. Longstreth, *City Center to Regional Mall,* esp. pp. 43–55.

16. Venturi, Scott Brown, and Izenour, *Learning from Las Vegas,* p. 20. Emphasis in the original.

17. Longstreth, *City Center to Regional Mall.*

18. Very little scholarly literature on mini-malls exists. Some scholars are begin-

ning to write about them, but the information here is taken from the files of the *Los Angeles Times*, especially, Judy Pasternak, "The Men of La Mancha" (September 28, 1986) in the *Los Angeles Times Magazine*; and James Rainey, "Mini-Mall Boom Hits a Dead End" (January 29, 1992). Also see, Greg Critser, "King of the Minimalls," *Los Angeles Magazine* 31 (1986), pp. 165–70.

19. Pasternak, "The Men of La Mancha," p. 25.

20. Ibid., p. 26.

21. James K. Skipper, Jr., and James E. Hughes, "Podiatry: A Medical Care Specialty in Quest of Full Professional Status and Recognition," in Rothstein, *Readings in American Healthcare*, p. 213.

22. This story, as well as other background information in this section, comes from Glenn Sonnedecker, *Kremers and Urdang's History of Pharmacy*, 4th ed. (Philadelphia: J. B. Lippincott, 1976), p. 291, in the chapter "Economic and Structural Development," which starts with a section titled "The Community Pharmacy."

23. For a quick overview of the history of alternative therapies, see Roy Porter, *Greatest Benefit to Mankind* (New York: W. W. Norton, 1997), pp. 389–96.

24. David M. Eisenberg, Roger B. Davis, Susan L. Eitner, Scott Appel, Sonja Wikey, Maria Van Rompay, and Ronald C. Kessler, "Trends in Alternative Medicine Use in the United States, 1990–1997," *JAMA* 280, no. 18 (November 11, 1998), pp. 1571–72.

25. Monmaney and Roan, "Hope or Hype," p. 1.

26. Shri Mishra, "Complementary/Alternative Medicine," in Heidi Sommer and Michael Dear, eds., *Health Atlas of Southern California* (Los Angeles: Southern California Studies Center, University of Southern California, 1999), pp. 29–30.

27. Arden G. Christen and Peter M. Pronych, *Painless Parker: A Dental Renegade's Fight to Make Advertising 'Ethical'"* (privately printed, 1995).

28. Regina Herzlinger, *Market-Driven Healthcare: Who Wins, Who Loses in the Transformation of America's Largest Service Industry* (Reading, Mass.: Addison-Wesley, 1997), pp. 33–36. The FTC's actions are discussed in Adam M. Friedman, "Comment: The Abandonment of the Antiquated Corporate Practices of Medicine Doctrine: Injecting a Dose of Efficiency into the Modern Health Care Environment," *Emory Law Journal* 47, no. 697 (Spring 1998).

29. McBride, *Integrating the City of Medicine*, p. 176. Also see, Vanessa Gamble, *The Black Community Hospital: Contemporary Dilemmas in Historical Perspective* (New York: Garland, 1989).

30. Don Lee, "An Anemic Rate of Health Coverage," *Los Angeles Times* (July 4, 1999).

31. Interview with Suzanne Sullivan, Vice President for Ambulatory Services at the University of California at San Francisco, November 20, 1998.

32. Ibid.

33. Eli Ginzberg, *Tomorrow's Hospital: A Look to the Twenty-First Century* (New Haven: Yale University Press, 1996), p. 40; National Center for Health Statistics, "Ambulatory Surgery in the United States, 1994," p. 1 for figures.

34. "ExecutiveChartbook: A Fight for Poor Eyes," *Hospitals and Health Networks* 72, no. 4 (1998), p. 68.

35. The decision raised considerable debate. For instance, Jonathan D. Moreno, "Out of Sight: Should Doctors Be Performing Eye Surgery in Shopping Malls?," found on the ABCNews.com web site on October 20, 1999. On changing surgical procedures, see Phil Connors, "Making the Cut: Surgery Should Become Less Invasive, Less Painful—and Maybe Even Less Expensive," *Wall Street Journal* (October 18, 1999), p. R11.

36. Rice, "Put Your Practice Where Shoppers Throng?" p. 140.

Epilogue: Orchestrating Healthcare

1. Quoted in Stephen Verderber and David J. Fine, *Healthcare Architecture in an Era of Radical Transformation* (New Haven: Yale University Press, 2000), p. 193.

2. Laura Green, "Build It, and They Might Come," *Hospitals and Health Networks* 70, no. 11 (June 5, 1996), pp. 51–54.

3. Christopher Press, "The Hospital as Airport," *Health Forum Journal* 42, no. 2 (March–April 1999), pp. 19–22.

4. Richard Saltus, "Losing Touch," *Boston Globe* (June 7, 1999), p. C1.

Selected Bibliography

This list only touches upon the huge literature on the relationship between architecture and the healthcare system, the evolution of cities, and commercial retailing. For a more extensive bibliography, please visit David Sloane's web site at the University of Southern California at http://www.usc.edu/sppd/mallmed.

Healthcare and Hospital

Burdett, Henry C. *Hospitals and Asylums of the World.* London: J. and A. Churchill, 1891–93.

Bynum, W. F., and Roy Porter, eds. *Companion Encyclopedia of the History of Medicine,* vol. 2. London: Routledge, 1993.

Davis, Michael Marks. *Clinics, Hospitals and Health Centers.* New York: Harper & Brothers, 1927.

Ginzberg, Eli. *Tomorrow's Hospital: A Look to the Twenty-First Century.* New Haven: Yale University Press, 1996.

Green, John. *City Hospitals.* Boston: Little, Brown, 1861.

Herzlinger, Regina E. *Market-Driven Healthcare: Who Wins, Who Loses in the Transformation of America's Largest Service Industry.* Reading, Mass.: Addison-Wesley, 1997.

Howell, Joel D. *Technology in the Hospital: Transforming Patient Care in the Early Twentieth Century.* Baltimore: Johns Hopkins University Press, 1995.

Illich, Ivan. *Medical Nemesis: The Expropriation of Health.* New York: Random House, 1976.

Long, Diane E., and Janet Golden, eds. *The American General Hospital: Communities and Social Contexts.* Ithaca, N.Y.: Cornell University Press, 1989.

Pascarelli, Emil F., ed. *Hospital-Based Ambulatory Care.* Norwalk, Conn.: Appleton-Century-Crofts, 1982.

Porter, Roy. *The Greatest Benefit to Mankind: A Medical History of Humanity*. New York: W. W. Norton, 1997.

Reverby, Susan, and David Rosner, eds. *Healthcare in America: Essays in Social History*. Philadelphia: Temple University Press, 1979.

Rosen, George. "The Hospital: Historical Sociology of a Community Institution." In Eliot Freidson, ed., *The Hospital in Modern Society*, pp. 1–36. New York: Free Press of Glencoe, 1963.

Rosenberg, Charles E. *The Care of Strangers: The Rise of America's Hospital System*. New York: Basic Books, 1987.

Rosner, David. *A Once Charitable Enterprise: Hospitals and Healthcare in Brooklyn and New York, 1885–1915*. Cambridge: Cambridge University Press, 1982.

Rothstein, William G., ed. *Readings in American Health Care: Current Issues in Socio-Historical Perspective*. Madison: University of Wisconsin Press, 1995.

Starr, Paul. *The Social Transformation of American Medicine: The Rise of a Sovereign Profession and the Making of a Vast Industry*. New York: Basic Books, 1982.

Stevens, Rosemary. *In Sickness and in Health: American Hospitals in the Twentieth Century*. New York: Basic Books, 1989.

Vogel, Morris J. *The Invention of the Modern Hospital: Boston, 1870–1930*. Chicago: University of Chicago Press, 1980.

Wylie, W. Gill. *Hospitals: Their History, Organization, and Construction*. New York: D. Appleton, 1877.

Look for further information in the *Bulletin of the History of Medicine* and the *Journal of the History of Medicine and Allied Professions*.

Healthcare Architecture

Adams, Annmarie. "Modernism and Medicine: The Hospitals of Stevens and Lee, 1916–1932." *Journal of the Society of Architectural Historians* 58, no. 1 (March 1999), pp. 42–61.

Billings, John Shaw. "Notes on Hospital Construction." *Public Health Reports and Papers of the American Public Health Association Meeting, 1874–75*. New York: Hurd & Houghton, 1876, pp. 385–88.

Brandt, Allan, and David C. Sloane. "Of Beds and Benches: Building the Modern American Hospital." In Peter Galison and Emily Thompson, eds., *The Architecture of Science*, pp. 281–308. Cambridge, Mass.: MIT Press, 1999.

Gaskie, Margaret. "Reinventing the Hospital." *Architectural Record* 173 (October 1985).

Green, Mitchel. "American Healthcare Design: Search for a New Image." *a+u* 201 (1987), pp. 102–9.

Hornsby, John Allan, and Richard E. Schmidt. *The Modern Hospital: Its Inspiration, Architecture, Equipment, Operation.* Philadelphia: W. B. Saunders, 1913.

Horsburgh, C. Robert, Jr. "Occasional Notes: Healing by Design." *The New England Journal of Medicine* 333 (September 14, 1995), pp. 735–40.

McKahan, Donald. "Healing by Design: Therapeutic Environments for Healthcare." *Interior Design* 64 (August 1993), pp. 108–9, 118.

Malkin, Jain. *Hospital Interior Architecture: Creating Healing Environments for Special Patient Populations.* New York: Van Nostrand Reinhold, 1992.

Miller, Richard L., and Earl S. Swensson. *New Directions in Hospital and Healthcare Facility Design.* New York: McGraw-Hill, 1995.

Pevsner, Nikolaus. *A History of Building Types.* Princeton, N.J.: Princeton University Press, 1976.

Podolsky, Doug. "Breaking Down the Walls: There's a Doctor in the Mall—and in the Barbershop, Too." *U.S. News and World Report* 121 (August 12, 1996), pp. 61–64.

Rosenfield, Isadore. *Hospitals: Integrated Design.* New York: Reinhold, 1951.

Sloane, David C. "Scientific Paragon to Hospital Mall: The Evolving Design of the Hospital, 1900–1990." *Journal of Architectural Education* 48, no. 2 (November 1994), pp. 82–98.

Stevens, Edward F. *The American Hospital of the Twentieth Century.* New York: Architectural Record Company, 1921.

Taylor, Jeremy. *The Architect and the Pavilion Hospital: Dialogue and Design Creativity in England, 1850–1914.* London: Leicester University Press, 1997.

Thompson, John D., and Grace Goldin. *The Hospital: A Social and Architectural History.* New Haven: Yale University Press, 1975.

Thompson, W. Gilman. "Modern Hospital Construction." *Journal of the American Medical Association* 49 (1907), pp. 993–99.

Verderber, Stephen, and David J. Fine. *Healthcare Architecture in an Era of Radical Transformation.* New Haven: Yale University Press, 2000.

Weathersby, William, Jr. "Easy Access: A 'Medical Mall' Plan Links a Diagnostic and Treatment Center with a Professional Building and Inpatient Bed Tower." *Hospitality Design* (May 1992), pp. 46–49.

Look for further information in *Architecture, Progressive Architecture,* and *Architectural Record.*

Urban Landscapes and Shopping Malls

Clausen, Meredith. "Shopping Centers." In J. Wilkes, ed., *Encyclopedia of Architecture: Design, Engineering, and Construction,* vol. 4, pp. 406–21. New York: John Wiley & Sons, 1989.

Davis, Timothy. "The Miracle Mile Revisited: Recycling, Renovation, and Simulation along the Commercial Strip." In Annmarie Adams and Sally McMurry, eds., *Exploring Everyday Landscapes: Perspectives in Vernacular Architecture*, vol. 7, pp. 93–114. Knoxville: University of Tennessee Press, 1997.

Gillette, Harold, Jr. "The Evolution of the Planned Shopping Center in Suburb and City." *Journal of American Planning Association* 51 (autumn 1985), pp. 449–60.

Groth, Paul. *Living Downtown: The History of Residential Hotels in the United States.* Berkeley: University of California Press, 1994.

Gruen, Victor. *The Heart of Our Cities, The Urban Crisis: Diagnosis and Cure.* New York: Simon and Schuster, 1964.

Hise, Greg. *Magnetic Los Angeles: Planning the Twentieth-Century Metropolis.* Baltimore: Johns Hopkins University Press, 1997.

Jackson, John Brinckerhoff. *Landscape in Sight: Looking at America.* Edited by Helen Lefkowitz Horowitz. New Haven: Yale University Press, 1997.

Jackson, Kenneth T. *Crabgrass Frontier: The Suburbanization of the United States.* New York: Oxford University Press, 1985.

Longstreth, Richard. *City Center to Regional Mall: Architecture, the Automobile, and Retailing in Los Angeles, 1920–1950.* Cambridge, Mass.: MIT Press, 1997.

Longstreth, Richard. *The Drive-in, the Supermarket, and the Transformation of Commercial Space in Los Angeles, 1914–1941.* Cambridge, Mass.: MIT Press, 1999.

Rowe, Peter. *Making a Middle Landscape.* Cambridge, Mass.: MIT Press, 1991.

Sloane, David C. *The Last Great Necessity: Cemeteries in American History.* Baltimore: Johns Hopkins University Press, 1991.

Sorkin, Michael. *Variations on a Theme Park: The New American City and the End of Public Space.* New York: Hill & Wang, 1992.

Upton, Dell. *Architecture in the United States.* New York: Oxford University Press, 1998.

Venturi, Robert, Denise Scott Brown, and Steven Izenour. *Learning from Las Vegas: The Forgotten Symbolism of Architectural Form.* Cambridge, Mass.: MIT Press, 1977.

Look for further information in the *Journal of Urban History* and the *Journal of the Society for Architectural History,* and from the Vernacular Architectural Forum, especially their wonderful Perspectives on Vernacular Architecture series.

Index

Page numbers in boldface type refer to illustrations.

195

About the Authors

DAVID CHARLES SLOANE is an associate professor in the School of Policy, Planning, and Development at the University of Southern California. Born in Youngstown, Ohio, he was raised in Syracuse, New York. He was trained at the University of Wisconsin and Syracuse University as an urban historian. He taught American history and the history of medicine at Dartmouth College and Medical School before moving to USC. He has published in the areas of cultural landscapes, history of medicine, and architectural and planning history, as well as contemporary issues in policing and communities and in community health planning. His book *The Last Great Necessity: Cemeteries in American History* (Johns Hopkins, 1991) was published as part of the *Creating the North American Landscape* series.

BEVERLIE CONANT SLOANE is a clinical associate professor in the Department of Family Medicine in the Keck School of Medicine at the University of Southern California. She was born in Norfolk, Virginia, and studied at Middlebury College, the University of Texas, and Syracuse University before accepting a position at Dartmouth College and Medical School. She pioneered peer education in techniques for treating HIV/AIDS and has published extensively on a wide range of health and medical issues. Her book *Partners in Health: Sexuality, Contraceptive, and Reproductive Health Issues,* first published in 1985, went through three editions.

Other Books in the Series

Land Between: Owens Valley, California
    REBECCA FISH EWAN

New York City's Washington Square
    EMILY KIES FOLPE

The Redrock Chronicles: Saving Wild Utah
    T. H. WATKINS

The Spaces between Buildings
    LARRY R. FORD